# Black...
# Care Essentials:
# Sports Medicine

# Blackwell's Primary Care Essentials Series

*Other books in Blackwell's Primary Care Essentials Series:*

*Blackwell's Primary Care Essentials: Cardiology*
John Sutherland

*Blackwell's Primary Care Essentials: Emergency Medicine*
Steven Diaz

*Blackwell's Primary Care Essentials: Gastrointestinal Disease*
David W. Hay

*Blackwell's Primary Care Essentials: Geriatrics, Second Edition*
Karen Gershman and Dennis M. McCullough

*Blackwell's Primary Care Essentials: Travel Medicine*
Robert P. Smith and Stephen D. Sears

*Blackwell's Primary Care Essentials: Urology*
Pamela Ellsworth and Stephen N. Rous

*Coming Soon:*

*Blackwell's Primary Care Essentials: Dermatology, Second Edition*
Stanford I. Lamberg

*Blackwell's Primary Care Essentials: Psychiatry, Second Edition*
David P. Moore

*Blackwell's Primary Care Essentials: Women's Health*
Amy Davis

# Blackwell's Primary Care Essentials: Sports Medicine

Thomas M. Howard, MD

*COL, MC, USA*
*Chief, Family Practice*
*Assistant Fellowship Director, Primary Care Sports Medicine*
*Fort Belvoir, Virginia*
*Assistant Professor of Family Medicine*
*Uniformed Services University of the Health Sciences*
*Bethesda, Maryland*

Janus D. Butcher, MD

*Department of Orthopedics and Sports Medicine*
*The Duluth Clinic*
*Clinical Assistant Professor*
*University of Minnesota School of Medicine*
*Duluth, Minnesota*

*Series Editor*

Daniel K. Onion, MD, MPH, FACP
*Professor of Community and Family Medicine*
*Dartmouth Medical School*
*Director of Maine-Dartmouth Family Practice Residency Program*
*Augusta, Maine*

**Blackwell**
**Science**

©2001 by Blackwell Science, Inc.

Editorial Offices:
Commerce Place, 350 Main Street, Malden, Massachusetts 02148, USA
Osney Mead, Oxford OX2 0EL, England
25 John Street, London WC1N 2BL, England
23 Ainslie Place, Edinburgh EH3 6AJ, Scotland
54 University Street, Carlton, Victoria 3053, Australia

*Other Editorial Offices:*
Blackwell Wissenschafts-Verlag GmbH, Kurfürstendamm 57, 10707 Berlin, Germany
Blackwell Science KK, MG Koden-macho Building, 7-10 Kodenmacho Nihombashi, Chuo-ku, Tokyo 104, Japan
Iowa State University Press, A Blackwell Science Company, 2121 S. State Avenue, Ames, Iowa 50014-8300, USA

*Distributors:*
*The Americas*
Blackwell Publishing
c/o AIDC
P.O. Box 20
50 Winter Sport Lane
Williston, VT 05495-0020
(Telephone orders: 800-216-2522; fax orders: 802-864-7626)

*Canada*
Login Brothers Book Company
324 Saulteaux Crescent
Winnipeg, Manitoba, R3J 3T2
(Telephone orders: 204-837-2987)

*Australia*
Blackwell Science Pty, Ltd.
54 University Street
Carlton, Victoria 3053
(Telephone orders: 03-9347-0300; fax orders: 03-9349-3016)

*Outside The Americas and Australia*
Blackwell Science, Ltd.
c/o Marston Book Services, Ltd.
P.O. Box 269
Abingdon
Oxon OX14 4YN
England
(Telephone orders: 44-01235-465500; fax orders: 44-01235-465555)

Library of Congress Cataloging-in-Publication Data

Howard, Thomas M.
   Blackwell's primary care essentials. Sports medicine / Thomas M. Howard, Janus Butcher.
      p.   cm. — (Blackwell's primary care essentials series)
   ISBN 0-86542-581-7
   1. Sports medicine—Handbooks, manuals, etc.  I. Butcher, Janus D.
   II. Blackwell Science.  III. Title.
   IV. Title: Sports medicine.  V. Series.
      [DNLM: 1. Athletic Injuries—Handbooks.   QT 29 H852b 2001]
   RC1211.H69 2001
   617.1'027—dc21

2001025051

Acquisitions: Nancy Anastasi Duffy
Development: Julia Casson
Production: Andover Publishing Services
Manufacturing: Lisa Flanagan
Marketing Manager: Toni Fournier
Cover design by Leslie Haimes
Typeset by Graphicraft Ltd., Hong Kong
Printed and bound by Capital City Press

Printed in the United States of America
01 02 03 04 5 4 3 2 1

The Blackwell Science logo is a trade mark of Blackwell Science Ltd., registered at the United Kingdom Trade Marks Registry

2254299X

# Contents

Contributors                                    xv
Preface                                         xvii
Medical Abbreviations                           xix
Journal Abbreviations                           xxvi

## Section I   GENERAL

1. OVERUSE INJURY AND STRESS FRACTURES          3
   Thomas Howard, MD and  David Brown, MD

   1.1 Overuse Injuries                         3
   1.2 Stress Fractures                         6


2. CORTICOSTEROID INJECTION THERAPY             9
   Janus Butcher, MD

   2.1  General Principles                      9
   2.2  Trigger Finger                          10
   2.3  De Quervain's Tenosynovitis             10
   2.4  TFCC                                    12
   2.5  Carpal Tunnel Syndrome                  13
   2.6  Tennis Elbow                            15
   2.7  Subacromial Space                       16
   2.8  Trochanteric Bursitis                   17
   2.9  Intra-articular Knee                    18
   2.10 Plantar Fascia                          19

3. ENVIRONMENTAL INJURIES   21
Neil Johnson, MD, Ted Epperley, MD,
and Brian Unwin, MD

3.1 Acute Mountain Sickness   21
3.2 HACE/HAPE   23
3.3 Trench Foot   25
3.4 Chilblains   26
3.5 Cold Urticaria   27
3.6 Frostbite   28
3.7 Hypothermia   30
3.8 Hyperthermia   34

4. NUTRITION AND ERGOGENICS   38
Koji Nishimura, MD and Thomas Howard, MD

4.1 Creatine   39
4.2 Anabolic Steroids   40
4.3 Human Growth Hormone   41
4.4 Erythropoietin   43
4.5 Stimulants   43

### Section II  ORTHOPEDIC PROBLEMS

5. CERVICAL SPINE INJURIES   49
John Glorioso, MD

5.1 Cervical Strain/Sprain   49
5.2 Cervical Spondylosis/Spinal Stenosis   50
5.3 Cervical Radiculopathy   51
5.4 Burner/Stinger   54
5.5 Cervical Instability   55

6. SHOULDER INJURIES   57
Thomas Howard, MD

6.1  AC Separation   57
6.2  Clavicle Fracture   58

| | | |
|---|---|---:|
| 6.3 | Anterior Shoulder Dislocation | 59 |
| 6.4 | Rotator Cuff Tear | 61 |
| 6.5 | AC Osteoarthritis | 65 |
| 6.6 | Shoulder Instability | 66 |
| 6.7 | Impingement and Subacromial Bursitis | 68 |
| 6.8 | Adhesive Capsulitis (Frozen Shoulder) | 70 |
| 6.9 | Rotator Cuff Tendinopathy | 71 |
| 6.10 | Biceps Tendonitis | 72 |
| 6.11 | Labral Tear | 74 |
| 6.12 | Calcific Bursitis and Tendonitis | 76 |

**7. ELBOW PROBLEMS**      77
Paul Pasquina, MD

| | | |
|---|---|---:|
| 7.1 | Lateral Epicondylitis (Tennis Elbow) | 77 |
| 7.2 | Medial Epicondylitis | 79 |
| 7.3 | PIN Entrapment | 81 |
| 7.4 | Olecranon Bursitis | 82 |
| 7.5 | Traumatic Elbow Injuries | 84 |
| 7.6 | MCL Instability | 85 |
| 7.7 | Distal Biceps Tendon Injuries | 87 |

**8. HAND INJURIES**      89
Wade Lillegard, MD

| | | |
|---|---|---:|
| 8.1 | Mallet Finger | 89 |
| 8.2 | Jersey Finger (Football Finger) | 90 |
| 8.3 | Boxer's Knuckle | 91 |
| 8.4 | Central Slip Avulsion | 92 |
| 8.5 | Trigger Finger | 93 |
| 8.6 | Collateral Ligament Tears | 94 |
| 8.7 | PIP Volar Plate Rupture | 95 |
| 8.8 | Skier's or Gamekeeper's Thumb | 96 |
| 8.9 | Middle Phalangeal Fracture | 97 |
| 8.10 | PIP Fracture Dislocation | 98 |
| 8.11 | Proximal Phalangeal Fractures | 99 |
| 8.12 | Metacarpal Fractures | 99 |
| 8.13 | Bennett's Fracture | 101 |

8.14 DIP Joint Dislocation ....... 101
8.15 PIP Dorsal Dislocation ....... 102
8.16 PIP Palmar Dislocation ....... 103
8.17 MCP Dislocation ....... 104

9. WRIST INJURIES ....... 106
Janus Butcher, MD

9.1 Scaphoid Fracture ....... 106
9.2 Hamate Fracture ....... 107
9.3 Kienböck's Disease ....... 108
9.4 Distal Radius Fracture ....... 109
9.5 De Quervain's Tenosynovitis ....... 111
9.6 Intersection Syndrome ....... 112
9.7 Extensor Carpi Ulnaris Tendinitis ....... 113
9.8 Flexor Tenosynovitis ....... 114
9.9 Common Extensor Tenosynovitis ....... 115
9.10 Scapholunate Dissociation ....... 116
9.11 TFCC Tear ....... 117
9.12 Dorsal Impaction Syndrome ....... 119
9.13 Wrist Ganglion ....... 119

10. BACK PROBLEMS ....... 121
Thomas Howard, MD

10.1 Mechanical Low Back Pain ....... 121
10.2 Discogenic Back Pain ....... 123
10.3 Sacroiliac Dysfunction ....... 125
10.4 Lumbar Spinal Stenosis ....... 127

11. HIP AND THIGH PROBLEMS ....... 130
Janus Butcher, MD

11.1 Femoral Stress Fracture ....... 130
11.2 Femoral Head AVN ....... 131
11.3 Acetabular Labral Tear ....... 132
11.4 Iliopectineal Bursitis ....... 133

| 11.5 | Adductor Tendon Strain | 134 |
| 11.6 | Iliopsoas Tendon Strain | 135 |
| 11.7 | Osteitis Pubis | 136 |
| 11.8 | Greater Trochanter Bursitis | 137 |
| 11.9 | Snapping Hip Syndrome | 139 |
| 11.10 | Hip Pointer | 139 |
| 11.11 | Piriformis Syndrome | 140 |
| 11.12 | Ischiogluteal Bursitis | 141 |
| 11.13 | Thigh Muscle Strains | 142 |
| 11.14 | Thigh Muscle Contusions | 143 |
| 11.15 | Myositis Ossificans | 144 |
| 11.16 | Avulsion Injuries | 145 |

## 12. KNEE PROBLEMS    146
Janus Butcher, MD

| 12.1 | ACL Tear | 146 |
| 12.2 | PCL Tear | 148 |
| 12.3 | Meniscus Injuries | 150 |
| 12.4 | Patellar Dislocation and Subluxation | 152 |
| 12.5 | Quadriceps/Patellar Tendon Rupture | 154 |
| 12.6 | MCL Tear | 155 |
| 12.7 | LCL Tear | 157 |
| 12.8 | Retropatellar Knee Pain | 158 |
| 12.9 | Quadriceps and Patellar Tendinitis | 160 |
| 12.10 | Medial Plica Syndrome | 161 |
| 12.11 | Prepatellar Bursitis | 162 |
| 12.12 | Pes Anserine Bursitis | 163 |
| 12.13 | Baker's Cysts | 164 |
| 12.14 | Iliotibial Band Friction Syndrome | 165 |

## 13. LEG PROBLEMS    167
Sean Mulvaney, MD and Francis O'Connor, MD

| 13.1 | Stress Fractures | 167 |
| 13.2 | Exertional Compartment Syndrome | 168 |
| 13.3 | Tennis Leg | 170 |
| 13.4 | Medial Tibial Stress Syndrome | 171 |

14. ANKLE INJURIES                                              172
     Sean Mulvaney, MD and Francis O'Connor, MD


     14.1   Lateral Ankle Sprain                                172
     14.2   Peroneal Tendon Subluxation and Dislocation         177
     14.3   High Ankle Sprain                                   178
     14.4   OCD                                                 180
     14.5   Achilles Tendon Rupture                             181
     14.6   Posterior Tendon Rupture                            183
     14.7   Anterolateral Soft-Tissue Impingement               184
     14.8   Posterior Tibialis Tendinopathy                     185
     14.9   Sinus Tarsi Syndrome                                186
     14.10  Distal Fibular Stress Fracture                      186
     14.11  Achilles Tendinopathy                               187


15. FOOT PROBLEMS                                               189
     Cathy Fieseler, MD


     15.1   Blisters                                            189
     15.2   Subungual Hematoma                                  190
     15.3   Hallux Valgus                                       190
     15.4   Turf Toe                                            191
     15.5   Hallux Rigidus                                      192
     15.6   Sesamoid Problems                                   192
     15.7   Morton's Neuroma                                    193
     15.8   Freiberg's Infarction                               194
     15.9   Phalangeal Fracture                                 195
     15.10  Metatarsal Fracture                                 195
     15.11  Metatarsal Stress Fracture                          196
     15.12  Fifth Metatarsal Fracture                           196
     15.13  Tarsal Stress Fracture                              197
     15.14  Lisfranc Fracture and Dislocation                   198
     15.15  Plantar Fasciitis                                   199
     15.16  Calcaneal Stress Fracture                           200
     15.17  Retrocalcaneal Bursitis                             201
     15.18  Tarsal Tunnel Syndrome                              201
     15.19  Os Trigonum Syndrome                                203

# Section III   MEDICAL PROBLEMS

16. NEUROLOGY                                         207
    Janus Butcher, MD

    16.1    Benign Exertional Headache              207
    16.2    Weightlifter's Headache                 208
    16.3    Exertional Migraine                     208
    16.4    Jogger's Migraine                       209
    16.5    Concussions                             210
    16.6    Second Impact Syndrome                  213
    16.7    Intracranial Hemorrhage                 213
    16.8    Carpal Tunnel Syndrome                  214
    16.9    Pronator Syndrome                       216
    16.10   Ulnar Nerve                             217
    16.11   Radial Tunnel Syndrome                  218


17. ADOLESCENT AND PEDIATRIC PROBLEMS               219
    Thomas Howard, MD and Harry McKinnon, MD

    17.1    Spondylolysis                           219
    17.2    Spondylolisthesis                       220
    17.3    Scheuermann's Kyphosis                  221
    17.4    OCD of the Knee                         222
    17.5    OCD of the Elbow                        224
    17.6    Osgood–Schlatter Disease                226
    17.7    Sinding–Larsen-Johansson                227
    17.8    Sever's Disease                         227
    17.9    Little League Elbow                     228
    17.10   Slipped Capital Femoral Epiphysis       230
    17.11   Legg–Calvé–Perthes                      231
    17.12   Toxic Synovitis of the Hip              232
    17.13   Salter–Harris Fractures                 232


18. CARDIOVASCULAR PROBLEMS                          235
    Robert Oh, MD and Charles Webb, MD

    18.1    Exercise-associated Collapse and Syncope   235
    18.2    Hypertension                            238

18.3 Hypertrophic Cardiomyopathy 241
18.4 Myocarditis 244
18.5 MVP 245
18.6 Long QT Syndrome 247

19. ISSUES UNIQUE TO THE FEMALE ATHLETE 248
Janus Butcher, MD

19.1 Exercise-associated Amenorrhea 248
19.2 Osteoporosis 250
19.3 Eating Disorders 251
19.4 Exercise in Pregnancy 253

20. GASTROINTESTINAL PROBLEMS 255
Janus Butcher, MD

20.1 Upper GI Symptoms 255
20.2 Lower GI Symptoms 257
20.3 GI Blood Loss 259
20.4 Hepatic Injury 261
20.5 Abdominal Pain (Side Stitch) 262

21. INFECTIOUS DISEASE 263
Thomas Howard, MD

21.1 Viral Syndrome 263
21.2 URI 264
21.3 Otitis Media 265
21.4 Sinusitis 266
21.5 Pneumonia 266
21.6 Infectious Mononucleosis 267
21.7 Diarrhea 268
21.8 Cellulitis 269
21.9 Herpes 270
21.10 Tinea 271

22. OTHER MEDICAL PROBLEMS                                    272
    Thomas Howard, MD and Harry McKinnon, MD

    22.1  Overtraining                                       272
    22.2  Exertional Rhabdomyolysis                          274
    22.3  Exercise-induced Hematuria                         275
    22.4  Exercise-induced Asthma                            276
    22.5  Exercise-induced Anaphylaxis                       278
    22.6  Cholinergic Urticaria                              280


INDEX                                                        281

# Notice

The indications and dosages of all drugs in this book have been recommended in the medical literature and conform to the practices of the general community. The medications described do not necessarily have specific approval by the Food and Drug Administration for use in the diseases and dosages for which they are recommended. The package insert for each drug should be consulted for use and dosage as approved by the FDA. Because standards for usage change, it is advisable to keep abreast of revised recommendations, particularly those concerning new drugs.

The views or assertions contained herein are the private views of the individual authors and are not to be construed as official or as reflecting the views of the Department of the Army or the Department of Defense.

# Contributors

David Brown, MD
MAJ, MC, USA
DeWitt Army Community
    Hospital
Fort Belvoir, Virginia

Janus D. Butcher, MD
The Duluth Clinic
Duluth, Minnesota

Ted Epperley, MD
COL, MC, USA
Eisenhower Army Medical Center
Fort Gordon, Georgia

Cathy Fieseler, MD
The Cleveland Clinic
Cleveland, Ohio

John Glorioso, MD
MAJ, MC, USA
Tripler Army Medical Center
Honolulu, Hawaii

Thomas M. Howard, MD
COL, MC, USA
DeWitt Army Community
    Hospital
Fort Belvoir, Virginia

Neil Johnson, MD
MAJ, MC, USA
Eisenhower Army Medical Center
Fort Gordon, Georgia

Wade Lillegard, MD
The Duluth Clinic
Duluth, Minnesota

Harry McKinnon, MD
MAJ, MC, USA
DeWitt Army Community
    Hospital
Fort Belvoir, Virginia

Sean Mulvaney, MD
CPT, MC, USA
Womack Army Medical Center
Fort Bragg, North Carolina

Koji Nishimura, MD
LTC, MC, USA
DeWitt Army Community
    Hospital
Fort Belvoir, Virginia

Francis G. O'Connor, MD
LTC, MC, USA
USUHS
Bethesda, Maryland

Robert Oh, MD
CPT, MC, USA
DeWitt Army Community
    Hospital
Fort Belvoir, Virginia

Paul Pasquina, MD
MAJ, MC, USA
Walter Reed Army Medical Center
Washington, D.C.

Brian Unwin, MD
LTC, MC, USA
Darnell Army Community
  Hospital
Fort Hood, Texas

Charles Webb, MD
CPT, MC, USA
Reynolds Army Community
  Hospital
Fort Sill, Oklahoma

# Preface

With the current emphasis on physical activity in children and adults, primary care providers are ever challenged with presentations of musculoskeletal and medical problems related to physical activity. The authors hope that this handbook will be a useful tool for all primary care providers (physicians, physician assistants, and nurse practioners) to carry in their coat pocket.

The authors remain ever grateful to the contributors for their time and expertise and to Blackwell Science and Dr. Dan Onion for this opportunity.

Thomas Howard, MD
Janus Butcher, MD

# Medical Abbreviations

| | |
|---|---|
| AAA | abdominal aortic aneurysm |
| AAS | acute abdominal series |
| AAT | anterior apprehension test |
| AC | acromio-clavicular |
| ACE | angiotensin converting enzyme |
| ACL | anterior cruciate ligament |
| ADAMS | aortic dilation and Marfan's syndrome |
| ADLs | activities of daily living |
| ADP | adenosine diphosphate |
| AI | aortic insufficiency |
| AITFL | anterior-inferior tibiofibular ligament |
| ALT | alanine aminotransferase |
| ANA | antinuclear antibody |
| AP | anterior-posterior |
| APMHR | age predicted maximum heart rate |
| ARDS | adult respiratory distress syndrome |
| asap | as soon as possible |
| ASCVD | arteriosclerotic cardiovascular disease |
| ASIS | anterior superior iliac spine |
| AST | aspartate aminotransferase |
| ATFL | anterior talofibular ligament |
| ATP | adenosine triphosphate |
| | |
| BCAA | branch chain amino acids |
| bcp's | birth control pills |
| BP | blood pressure |
| BPD | bipolar disorder |
| BUN | blood urea nitrogen |
| bw | body weight |
| | |
| CAD | coronary artery disease |
| CAM | brand name of removable short-leg walking boot |

| | |
|---|---|
| CBC | complete blood count |
| CFL | calcaneofibular ligament |
| CHF | congestive heart failure |
| CMC | carpal-metacarpal |
| CP | creatine phosphate |
| CPK | creatine phosphokinase |
| CR | creatinine |
| CRP | creactive protein |
| CSF | cerebrospinal fluid |
| CT | computed tomography |
| CTS | carpal tunnel syndrome |
| CV | cardiovascular |
| CVA | cerebrovascular accident |
| CVD | cardiovascular disease |
| CXR | chest x-ray |
| | |
| dbl | dreaded black line |
| DEXA | dual energy x-ray absorptiometry |
| DF | dorsiflexion |
| DIC | disseminated intravascular coagulation |
| DIP | distal interphalangeal |
| DISI | dorsal intercalated segment instability |
| DJD | degenerative joint disease |
| DM | diabetes mellitus |
| DRUJ | distal radioulnar joint |
| DTR | deep tendon reflex |
| DVT | deep vein thrombosis |
| | |
| EAA | exercise-associated amenorrhea |
| EAC | exercise-associated collapse, or external auditory canal |
| EBV | Epstein-Barr virus |
| ECHO | echocardiogram |
| ECRB | extensor carpi radialis brevis |
| ECS | exertional compartment syndrome |
| ECU | extensor carpi ulnaris |
| EDV | end diastolic volume |
| EEG | electroencephalogram |
| EDC | extensor digitorum communis |
| EGD | esophago-gastro-duodenoscopy (aka endoscopy) |
| EHL | extensor hallucis longus |

| | |
|---|---|
| EKG | electrocardiogram |
| EMG | electromyogram |
| EP | electrophysiologic |
| EPL | extensor pollicis longus |
| EPO | erythropoietin |
| ER | external rotators |
| ESI | epidural steroid injection |
| ESR | erythrocyte sedimentation rate |
| ETOH | ethanol |
| EV | eversion |
| | |
| FABER | Flexion **AB**duction External **R**otation |
| FCU | flexor carpi ulnaris |
| FD | flexor digitorum |
| FDP | flexor digitorum profundus |
| FH | flexor hallucis |
| fhx | family history |
| FSH | follicle stimulating hormone |
| FVC | forced vital capacity |
| fx | fracture |
| | |
| GABS | Group A beta-hemolytic streptococcus |
| gc | gonorrhea |
| GGT | gamma-glutamyl transpeptidase |
| GH | glenohumeral |
| GI | gastrointestinal |
| GNRH | gonadotropin releasing hormone |
| gxt | Graded Exercise Test |
| | |
| HCG | human chorionic gonadotropin |
| HCM | hypertrophic cardiomyopathy |
| HDL | high-density lipoprotein |
| hep | hepatitis |
| HGH | human growth hormone |
| 5-HIAA | 5-hydroxyindoleacetic acid |
| HIV | human immunodeficiency virus |
| HNP | herniated nucleus pulposus |
| HPA | hypothalamic-pituitary axis |
| h/o | history of |
| hr | heart rate |

| | |
|---|---|
| hrr | heart rate reserve |
| HTN | hypertension |
| hx | history |
| | |
| IBD | inflammatory bowel disease |
| IBS | irritable bowel syndrome |
| ibw | ideal body weight |
| ICD | implantable cardiac defibrillator |
| IDT | Inferior Dislocation Test |
| ILGF-1 | insulin-like growth factor |
| im | intramuscular |
| IOC | International Olympic Committee |
| IOM | interosseous membrane |
| IP | interphalangeal |
| ir | internal rotation |
| IT | iliotibial |
| ITB | iliotibial band |
| iv | intravenous |
| | |
| JRA | juvenile rheumatoid arthritis |
| | |
| KOH | potassium hydroxide |
| | |
| lat | lateral |
| LBP | low back pain |
| LCL | lateral collateral ligament |
| LCP | Legg-Calvé Perthes |
| LDH | lactate dehydrogenase |
| LDL | low-density lipoproteins |
| le | lower extremity |
| LES | lower esophageal sphincter |
| LFTs | liver function tests |
| LH | luteinizing hormone |
| LQTS | long QT syndrome |
| LT | lunotriquetral |
| LVH | left ventricular hypertrophy |
| | |
| mc | metacarpal |
| MCL | medial collateral ligament |

| | |
|---|---|
| MCP | metacarpal-phalangeal |
| MI | myocardial infarction; or mitral insufficiency |
| MO | myositis ossificans |
| MR | mitral regurgitation |
| MRI | magnetic resonance imaging |
| mtp | metatarsal-phalangeal |
| MTSS | medial tibial stress syndrome |
| MVA | motor vehicle accident |
| MVP | mitral valve prolapse |
| | |
| NCAA | National Collegiate Athletic Association |
| NCS | nerve conduction study |
| NCV | nerve conduction velocities |
| NIH | National Institutes of Health |
| NSAID | non-steroidal anti-inflammatory drug |
| | |
| $O_2$ | oxygen |
| OA | osteoarthritis |
| OCD | osteochondral defect or osteochondritis dessicans |
| OCL | osteochondral lesion |
| OMT | osteopathic manipulative therapy |
| ORIF | operative reduction and internal fixation |
| OTC | over-the-counter |
| | |
| PCL | posterior cruciate ligament |
| $PCO_2$ | partial pressure of carbon dioxide |
| PDT | posterior dislocation test |
| PE | pulmonary embolism |
| PF | plantarflexion or palmarflexion |
| PIN | posterior interosseous nerve |
| PIP | proximal interphalangeal |
| PITFL | posterior-inferior tibiofibular ligament |
| PMN | polymorphonuclear neutrophils |
| PPE | preparticipation physical exam |
| PRICEMM | protect, rest, ice, compression, elevation, medications, modalities |
| PTFL | posterior talofibular ligaments |
| PUD | peptic ulcer disease |

| | |
|---|---|
| qid | 4 times a day |
| q2h | every 2 hours |
| QT | QT interval of QRS complex |
| | |
| RA | rheumatoid arthritis |
| RBC | red blood cell |
| RC | rotator cuff |
| RDA | recommended daily allowance |
| rEPO | recombinant erythropoietin |
| RF | rheumatoid factor |
| ROM | range of motion |
| r/o | rule out |
| RPPS | retropatellar pain syndrome |
| RV | right ventricle |
| RVH | right ventricular hypertrophy |
| | |
| SAH | subarachnoid hemorrhage |
| SBE | subacute bacterial endocarditis |
| SCFE | slipped capital femoral epiphysis |
| SGOT | *see* AST |
| SI | sacroiliac |
| SITS | Supraspinatus, Infraspinatus, Teres Minor, Subscapularis |
| SLAP | superior labral anterior-posterior |
| SLJ | Sinding-Larsen-Johansson disease |
| SPECT | single-photon emission computed tomography |
| sq | subcutaneous |
| SSRI | selective serotonin reuptake inhibitor |
| STD | sexually transmitted disease |
| SV | stroke volume |
| | |
| TCA | tricyclic antidepressant |
| TENS | transcutaneous electrical nerve stimulation |
| TFCC | triangular fibrocartilage complex |
| TIA | transient ischemic attack |
| tid | 3 times a day |
| TLSO | thoraco-lumbar spinal orthosis |
| TM | tympanic membrane |
| TMJ | temporal mandibular joint |
| TSH | thyroid stimulating hormone |
| TTP | tenderness to palpation |

| UA | urinalysis |
| UCL | ulnar collateral ligament |
| UTI | urinary tract infection |
| | |
| VISI | volar intercalated segment instability |
| VMA | vanillylmandelic acid |
| VMO | vastus medialis obliquus |
| $VO_2max$ | maximal oxygen consumption |
| | |
| WBC | white blood cells, or white blood count |
| WPW | Wolff-Parkinson-White syndrome |
| | |
| xc | cross-country |

# Journal Abbreviations

| | |
|---|---|
| AAOS Instr Course Lect | American Academy of Orthopedic Surgery Instruction Course Lectures |
| Acta Orthop Scand | Acta Orthopedia Scandinavia |
| Am Fam Phys | American Family Physician |
| Am J Gastroenterol | American Journal of Gastroenterology |
| Am J Knee Surg | American Journal of Knee Surgery |
| Am J Sports Med | American Journal of Sports Medicine |
| Ann Emerg Med | Annals of Emergency Medicine |
| Ann Inter Med | Annals of Internal Medicine |
| Arch Fam Med | Archives of Family Medicine |
| Arch Intern Med | Archives of Internal Medicine |
| Aust J Sci Med | Australia Journal of Science Medicine |
| Br J Sports Medicine | British Journal of Sports Medicine |
| Cardio Clin | Cardiology Clinics |
| Clin J Sport Med | Clinical Journal of Sports Medicine |
| Clin Sport Med | Clinics in Sports Medicine |
| Crit Care Clin | Critical Care Clinics |
| Curr Opin Rheumatol | Current Opinions in Rheumatology |
| Dig Dis Sci | Digestive Disease Science |
| Exerc Sport Sci Rev | Exercise and Sport Sciences Reviews |
| Geriatrics | Geriatrics |
| GSSI Sports Sci Ex | Gatorade Sports Science Institute Sports Science Exchange |
| Int J Sports Med | International Journal of Sports Medicine |
| J Accid Emerg Med | Journal of Accident and Emergency Medicine |

| | |
|---|---|
| J Am Acad Dermatol | Journal of the American Academy of Dermatology |
| J Am Acad Orthop Sug | Journal of the American Academy of Orthopedic Surgery |
| J Anat | Journal of Anatomy |
| J Appl Physiol | Journal of Applied Physiology |
| J Clin Endo and Met | Journal of Clinical Endocrinology and Metabolism |
| J Hand Surg | Journal of Hand Surgery |
| J of All and Clin Imm | Journal of Allergy and Clinical Immunology |
| J Rheumatol | Journal of Rheumatology |
| J Trauma | Journal of Trauma |
| JBJS | Journal of Bone and Joint Surgery |
| Mayo Clin Proc | Mayo Clinical Proceedings |
| Med Clin N Amer | Medical Clinics of North America |
| Med Sci Sports Exerc | Medicine and Science in Sports and Exercise |
| N Z Med | New Zealand Journal of Medicine |
| NEJM | New England Journal of Medicine |
| Neurol Clin | Neurology Clinics |
| Nut Aspects of Ex | Nutritional Aspects of Exercise |
| Ortho Clin North Am | Orthopedic Clinics of North America |
| Orthopedic Sports Med | *Orthopedic Sports Medicine* |
| Ped Clin No Am | Pediatric Clinics of North America |
| Ped Rev | Pediatric Review |
| Phy Sportmed | The Physician and Sportsmedicine |
| Skeletal Radiol | Skeletal Radiology |
| Surg Clin North Amer | Surgical Clinics of North America |

# Section I

# GENERAL

# 1 Overuse Injury and Stress Fractures

## 1.1 OVERUSE INJURIES

Exerc Sport Sci Rev 1992;20:99; Phy Sportmed 1997;25(5):88

**Cause:** Inadequate recovery from training or too much, too soon, too fast

**Epidem:** 30–50% of all sports injuries; twice as frequent as traumatic injuries

**Pathophys:**

- Normal "adaptive response" of tissue to overload

  *Local inflammation*—acute macro or microtraumatic injury with local bleeding/clot, release of chemotactic cytokines, and invasion of PMNs and monocytes

  *Reparative*—monocytes differentiate to macrophages and fibroblasts with stimulation of neovascularization and establishment of initial collagen matrix

  *Remodeling/strengthening*—organization of extracellular matrix and fibroblasts and reduction of immature cells (usually 4 months)

- Repetitive microtrauma from tissue overload with inadequate recovery or impaired tissue healing

- Principle of transition with change in mode, intensity, duration, equipment, or other with a mismatch of overload and recovery

- Intrinsic factors (unique to the individual)

  Malalignment

  Muscle imbalance

  Inflexibility

  Weakness

  Joint instability

- Extrinsic factors
  - Training errors
  - Equipment
  - Technique
  - Environment
  - Sports acquired deficiencies (weakness, inflexibility, etc.)
- A common term used for these chronic conditions is tendinopathy or tendinosis implying that the "chronic tendinitis" is more a degenerative process (Clin J Sport Med 1998;8:151)
  - On histology, the tendon will appear as disorganized fibroblasts and neovascularization, implying inadequate or deranged adaptive response

**Sx:**

- Pain
  - Nirschl's Pain Phase Scale (Phy Sportmed 1997;25(5):88)
  - *Phase 1*—stiffness or pain after activity; resolved in 24 hrs
  - *Phase 2*—stiffness or mild soreness before activity relieved by warm-up; not present with activity but returning afterward and lasting up to 48 hrs
  - *Phase 3*—stiffness or mild soreness before activity partially relieved by warm-up and minimally present during activity, but not altering activity
  - *Phase 4*—more intense than phase 3 causing alteration in activity and occurs with ADLs, but not altering ADLs
  - *Phase 5*—significant pain before, during, and after activity causing alteration of activity; pain with ADLs, but not altering them
  - *Phase 6*—phase 5 pain that persists even with complete rest; pain limits performance of ADLs and household chores
  - *Phase 7*—phase 6 pain that disrupts sleep and intensifies with activity
- Performance decrements
- h/o transition or overload in training

**Si:**

- Soft tissue or bony tenderness
- Evidence of inflammation
- Weakness and muscle imbalance
- Inflexibility
- Biomechanical deficiencies
- Examine one joint proximal and distal

- Examine the entire kinetic chain, i.e., the entire leg in a runner or the upper and lower back and LE flexibility in a thrower or tennis player
- Deficiencies in parts of this kinetic chain that helps us generate sport-specific movement usually overload more distal structures, i.e., shoulder weakness and dysfunction contributing to medial or lateral tennis elbow

**Crs:** If not addressed continued poor performance and pain

**Cmplc:** Stress fx; chronic tendinopathy; tendon/muscle rupture

**DiffDx:** See individual musculoskeletal chapters

**Xray:**
- Plain films—to eval for occult tumor, degeneration or heterotopic calcifications
- CT—effective for evaluating bone for tumor or fracture; further eval of soft tissues enhanced by intra-articular contrast
- MRI—best technique to visualize soft tissues to see degeneration, tear, tendinopathy, or inflammation

**Rx:**

Most providers use the mnemonic PRICEMM to organize their management (Protect, Rest, Ice, Compression, Elevation, Medications, Modalities)

- Make a pathoanatomic diagnosis (see individual chapters)
- Control inflammation

  *Post injury or activity ice*—ice massage (or application of a frozen bag of peas or corn) 15 min as frequent as q2h if necessary

  *NSAIDs*—traditional NSAIDs (Advil, Aleve, Motrin, Naprosyn, etc.) or COX-2 inhibitors (Vioxx or Celebrex)

  Consider oral or injected steroids in some cases

  *Relative rest*—avoid the offending activity; maintain ROM, cross training to maintain motion and central aerobics without continuing to reproduce the injury

- Promote healing

  Rehabilitate to recover strength, endurance and flexibility, and balance between agonist and antagonist muscle groups

- Increase fitness

  Central fitness through cross training

- Control abuse

  Proper equipment (shoes, racquet, club, shaft, etc.)

Establish a new training program that allows recovery time
*Technique*—consider lesions, instruction, coaching
Taping and bracing
- Return to activity
  Full pain-free ROM
  85% strength
- Adequate psychologic recovery
  Stages of psychologic recovery include shock, realization, mourning, acknowledgement, coping, and setting minor and major goals

## 1.2 STRESS FRACTURES

Clin Sports Med 1997;16:339; Am Fam Phys 1997;56:175; Ortho Clin North Am 1995;26:423; Am J Sports Med 1987;15:46.

**Cause:** Repetitive loading of bone unaccustomed to such stresses; overtraining. Contributing role of nutritional and hormonal factors (e.g., female athlete triad)

**Epidem:** Difficult to assess actual incidence due to variations in definition and diagnostic modality applied (i.e., hx/PE vs. plain films vs. bone scan). Military population studies—yearly incidence 2% in males and 11.8% in females (J Military Med 1983;148:666). Large review over last 10–15 years 0.9–3.2% in males and 3.49–21% in females (Ex Sports Sci Rev 1989;17:379). Athletic population studies—general incidence 3.7%, with 2% per year in men and 6.9% per year for women (Am J Sports Med 1994;22:248).

**Pathophys:** Increased activity dose outstrips a bone's ability to adapt. An inappropriate increase in frequency, duration, and intensity of exercise + negative modulators (e.g., hormonal deficiency, inadequate nutrition) predispose to injury. Repetitive stress causes periosteal resorption >> remodeling leading to cortical weakening. Spectrum of injury ranges from stress response to complete fracture.

**Sx:** Insidious onset of exertional bone pain occurring at progressively lower workloads. Progresses from mild to severe pain over days to weeks. Initially only affects sporting activity but if injury is not addressed pain may be present with ADLs.

**Si:** PE may be completely unrevealing. May have focal tenderness, induration, edema, and warmth. For long bone stress fx, percussion or application of a tuning fork at a distance from the symptomatic site may cause pain at the fx site.

**Cmplc:** Complete fracture. Delayed on nonunion at high-risk sites. Avascular necrosis (femoral head).

**DiffDx:** Chronic soft tissue injury (e.g., tendonitis, muscle strain, etc.), exertional compartment syndrome (see 13.2), medial tibial stress syndrome (see 13.4), degenerative joint disease, infection, and tumor (e.g., osteoid osteoma, osteoblastoma, eosinophilic granuloma, osteosarcoma, metastatic carcinomas).

**Lab:** Largely noncontributory. CBC and ESR if indicated.

**Xray:**
- Site-specific radiographs may reveal periosteal new bone with sclerosis or a radiolucent line (the "dreaded black line") as early as 3 weeks but may not have changes for up to 3 months. Poor sensitivity (30%) but highly specific if positive. CT scans are often nonspecific and are considered less sensitive than plain films because fracture lines are not visualized in all cases
- Technesium-99 three-phase (current "gold standard" for stress fx diagnosis) single–phase bone scan or SPECT scan can show changes as early as 48–72 hours. For patients under 65, nearly 100% sensitive and in patients over age 65, 80–95% sensitive. Remains positive from 6 months to 2 years out from injury
- Emerging role of extremity-dedicated MRI. Already the imaging study of choice for patients with femoral neck and pelvic fractures that have normal plain films but a high clinical suspicion for injury. Limited screening protocols and edema-sensitive sequences are increasing MRI's cost-effectiveness compared to other modalities

**Rx:**

*Prevention:* Allow bone adequate time for an adaptive response by applying cyclic training program alternating with periods of rest. Emphasis on cross training with activities that reduce or eliminate ground-reactive forces (e.g., using stair climbing/elliptical training machines, cycling, swimming, and pool running). Maintain adequate caloric and calcium intake. Especially be aware of the female athlete triad and use hormonal replacement therapy if indicated.

*Rehabilitation:* Phase I
- Rest from offending/painful activity
- Address nutritional and hormonal risk factors
- Crutches if necessary for short period until ADLs pain free
- NSAIDs/ice
- Stretching/flexibility exercises
- Cross train for 6 weeks to maintain cardiovascular fitness
- If no pain, progress to phase II
- If pain still present at 6 weeks check for propagation on plain films
  If no progression on xrays can start cyclic progression
  If there is progression on xrays, repeat phase I

Phase II
- Cyclic progression
- Gradual re-introduction to sport-specific activities
- Return to sports

*Referral:* Any bone involvement where complete fracture would have serious complications
- Tibia—mid-shaft or anterior cortical involvement (see 13.1)
- Tarsal navicular (see 15.13)
- Fifth metatarsal (Jones fx) (see 15.12)
- Femoral neck—superior cortex especially prone to displacement (see 11.1)
- Spine—compression fractures
- Any injury where conservative management has yielded an inadequate response; persistent pain/limitation in activity; progression of injury on follow-up imaging
- Any elite athlete where more rapid rehabilitation and return to play is required

**Return to Activity:**
Usual time period for return to sports participation (wk):
- Femoral
  Neck—7.5–11.5
  Shaft—8–14
- Tibia—6–12
- Fibula—6
- Tarsal navicular—16–20
- Metatarsal—6–12
- Pubic rami—8–20

# 2 Corticosteroid Injection Therapy

Clin Sport Med 1995;14:353; Geriatrics 1990;45:45; Curr Opin
Rheumatol 1999;11:417

## 2.1 GENERAL PRINCIPLES

**Medications:**
- Betamethasone acetate (Celestone Soluspan) 6 mg/cc
- Dexamethasone acetate (Decadron LA) 8 mg/cc
- Triamcinolone diacetate (Aristocort) 40 mg/cc
- Local anesthetics: lidocaine 1%, bupivacaine 0.25%

**Mode of Action/Effects:**
- Inhibit prostaglandin synthesis, and release of cytokines, and other chemical mediators of the inflammatory cascade
- Inhibit activation and function of neutrophils, macrophages, fibroblasts, and basophils
- Major result is diminished pain and reduced soft tissue swelling

**General Side Effects/Complications:**
- Local effects and complications: infection (very low risk with proper technique), nerve injury, pneumothorax, subcutaneous fat atrophy, skin color changes
- Allergic reactions: anesthetic or corticosteroid preparation
- Tendon and joint complications: tendon rupture, articular cartilage damage, and osteoporosis
- Other reactions: steroid flare (2% of injections), vasovagal response (most common with upper extremity injections)
- Diabetes mellitus: hyperglycemia

- Glaucoma: reported potential complication. Rare in practice
- Some studies suggest may actually inhibit healing and lead to (transient) weakening of soft tissues

**Contraindications:**
- Acute systemic infection, joint infection, or cellulitis at injection site
- Poorly controlled diabetes
- History of reaction to any components of injection solution
- Injection into a prosthetic joint or fracture site

## 2.2 TRIGGER FINGER

**Indication:**
- Painful catching or locking of finger with active flexion

**Anatomy:**
- Flexor tendon nodule typically just proximal to MCP joint
- Will translate with active flexion/extension of the affected digit

**Procedure:**
- Using a $^5/_8$ in. 25-gauge needle instill solution into flexor tendon sheath at the palpable nodule (Figure 2.1)

**Medication:**
- $^3/_4$ cc betamethasone (Celestone 6 mg/cc) in $^1/_4$ cc lidocaine (1%)
- $^3/_4$ cc triamcinolone (40 mg/cc) in $^1/_4$ cc lidocaine (1%)

**Precautions:**
- Ensure that pain is not the result of infectious flexor tenosynovitis
- Avoid injection into subcutaneous fat (may cause fat atrophy)

## 2.3 DE QUERVAIN'S TENOSYNOVITIS

**Indication:**
- Reduce pain in extensor pollicis brevis and abductor pollicis to allow adequate rehabilitation and tissue healing

**Anatomy:**
- EPB and abductor pollicis tendons contained in 1st dorsal wrist compartment
- Tendons form the dorsal and volar boundaries of the anatomic snuff box

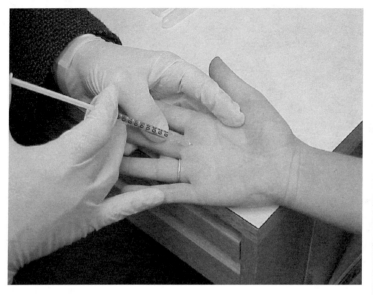

**Figure 2.1.** Trigger finger injection

Procedure:
- 25-gauge $1^1/_2$ in. needle is inserted at the anatomic snuffbox into the 1st dorsal wrist compartment directed proximally (Figure 2.2)

Medication:
- 1–2 cc betamethasone (Celestone 6 mg/cc) in 3 cc lidocaine (1%)
- 1–2 cc triamcinolone (40 mg/cc) in 3 cc lidocaine (1%)

Precautions:
- Avoid injection into subcutaneous fat (may cause fat atrophy)
- Superficial injection may cause skin discoloration

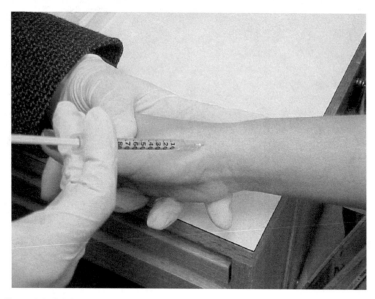

**Figure 2.2.** De Quervain's tenosynovitis injection

## 2.4 TRIANGULAR FIBROCARTILAGE COMPLEX (TFCC)

Indication:
- Chronic ulnar sided wrist pain due to tear or degeneration of the TFCC

Anatomy:
- TFCC fills the space between the distal ulna (ulnar styloid) and proximal medial carpus

Procedure:
- After sterile prep, solution is injected through a 1¹/₂ in. 25-gauge needle via a medial approach. The needle is inserted just distal to the ulnar styloid (Figure 2.3)

Medication:
- 1–2 cc betamethasone (Celestone 6 mg/cc) in 3 cc lidocaine (1%)
- 1–2 cc triamcinolone (40 mg/cc) in 3 cc lidocaine (1%)

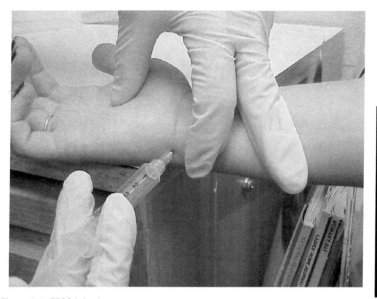

**Figure 2.3.** TFCC injection

Precautions:
- Avoid injection into subcutaneous fat (may cause fat atrophy)
- Superficial injection may cause skin discoloration

## 2.5 CARPAL TUNNEL SYNDROME

Indication:
- Reduction of flexor tendon inflammation to reduce pain and median nerve compression

Anatomy:
- Carpal tunnel formed by the carpal bones and flexor retinaculum
- Contains flexor digitorum profundus and superficialis, flexor pollicis longus, flexor carpi radialis, and the median nerve

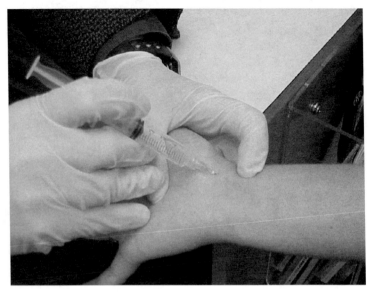

**Figure 2.4.** Carpal tunnel injection

**Procedure:**
- After sterile prep, a 1¹/₂ in. 25-gauge needle is placed beneath the flexor retinaculum at the radial border of the palmaris longus at the distal flexor crease. Needle is directed at an approximately 45-degree angle proximally (Figure 2.4)

**Medication:**
- 1–2 cc betamethasone (Celestone 6 mg/cc) in 1 cc lidocaine (1%)
- 1–2 cc triamcinolone (40 mg/cc) in 1 cc lidocaine (1%)

**Precautions:**
- Avoid injection into subcutaneous fat (may cause fat atrophy)
- Superficial injection may cause skin discoloration
- Avoid injection into median nerve (patient will complain of pain shooting into hand)
- Relapse of symptoms very common shortly after injection

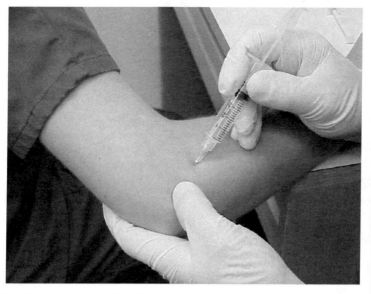

**Figure 2.5.** Lateral tennis elbow injection

## 2.6 TENNIS ELBOW

Indication:
  • Tenderness at origin of ECRB tendon on lateral epicondyle
Anatomy:
  • Common extensor tendon (extensor carpi radialis brevis, extensor digitorum, extensor digiti minimi, extensor carpi ulnaris) origin at the lateral epicondyle
Procedure:
  • After sterile prep, solution is injected in a wide pattern along the insertion of the extensor tendons (Figure 2.5)
Medication:
  • 1–2 cc betamethasone (Celestone 6 mg/cc) in 3 cc lidocaine (1%)
  • 1–2 cc triamcinolone (40 mg/cc) in 3 cc lidocaine (1%)
Precautions:
  • Avoid injection into subcutaneous fat (may cause fat atrophy)
  • Superficial injection may cause skin discoloration

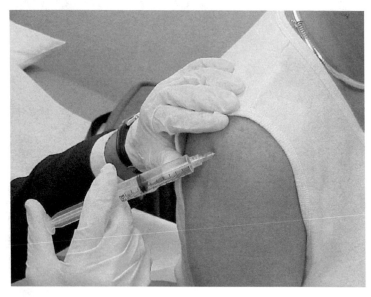

**Figure 2.6.** Shoulder subacromial space injection

## 2.7 SUBACROMIAL SPACE

Indication:
- Reduction of pain due to inflammation of supraspinatus tendon, subacromial bursa, or lateral impingement

Anatomy:
- Subacromial space formed by acromial arch (acromion and coraco-acromial ligament) superolaterally, supraspinatus muscle inferiorly, clavicle anteriorly, and the spine of the scapula posteriorly
- Potential space occupied by subacromial bursa

Procedure:
- After sterile prep, $1\frac{1}{2}$ in. 25-gauge needle is introduced at the posterolateral shoulder (junction of the posterior and middle deltoid muscle), just below the acromion. Needle should be parallel to the floor and directed toward the AC joint (Figure 2.6)

Medication:
- 1–2 cc betamethasone (Celestone 6 mg/cc) in 7–8 cc lidocaine (1%)
- 1–2 cc triamcinolone (40 mg/cc) in 7–8 cc lidocaine (1%)

Precautions:
- Avoid injection into subcutaneous fat (may cause fat atrophy)
- Superficial injection may cause skin discoloration

## 2.8 TROCHANTERIC BURSITIS

Indication:
- Pain relief to allow participation in physical therapy, exercise, and continued ADLs

Anatomy:
- Up to three separate bursae along the superior margin of the greater trochanter and are found between the iliotibial band (ITB) and trochanter.

Procedure:
- After sterile prep, palpate the soft tissue at the superior margin of the trochanter to identify the points of maximal tenderness. Insert a 2 in. or longer, 25-gauge needle and inject solution as the needle is withdrawn. The bursa is irritated transiently by the anesthetic and will reproduce the patient's symptoms. The remainder of the solution is injected at this point

Medication:
- 2–3 cc betamethasone (Celestone 6 mg/cc) in 10 cc lidocaine (1%)
- 2–3 cc triamcinolone (40 mg/cc) in 10 cc lidocaine (1%)

Precautions:
- Sciatic nerve lies deep and posterior to the trochanter
- If bony contact is made (femoral neck), the injection will be intra-articular

## 2.9 INTRA-ARTICULAR KNEE

**Indication:**
- Relief of pain due to degenerative joint disease, subacute meniscal tear, or patellofemoral dysfunction

**Anatomy:**
- Joint formed by articulation of tibia, femur, and patella. Continuous space from suprapatellar pouch to patellar tendon insertion

**Procedure:**
- Multiple approaches possible. Knee should be thoroughly prepped with betadine and sterile techniques employed
- Anterior approach: with the patient sitting and the knee flexed 90 degrees, a $1^1/_2$ in. 25-gauge needle is inserted on either the lateral or medial border of patellar tendon. The needle is directed directly into the notch and the solution is injected into the notch
- Lateral suprapatellar approach: with patient supine, the superior lateral margin of the patella is palpated and a 25-gauge needle is inserted below the patella. The solution is instilled at this point. This approach is also used for aspiration. A 22-gauge needle is inserted in a similar fashion. Aspiration is accomplished with a 60-cc syringe. The aspiration syringe may then be replaced with the syringe containing the steroid solution and the injection accomplished through the same needle (Figure 2.7)

**Medication:**
- 1–2 cc betamethasone (Celestone 6 mg/cc) in 7–8 cc lidocaine (1%)
- 1–2 cc triamcinolone (40 mg/cc) in 7–8 cc lidocaine (1%)

**Precautions:**
- Avoid injection through meniscus as this is quite painful
- Limit injections to 2 to 3 injections in 12 month period; repetitive injection can lead to softening of cartilage and further damage
- Avoid injection into subcutaneous fat (may cause fat atrophy)
- Superficial injection may cause skin discoloration

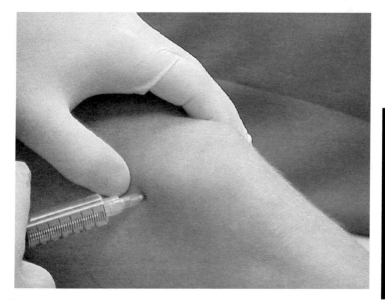

**Figure 2.7.** Intra-articular knee injection

## 2.10 PLANTAR FASCIA

Indication:
- Relief of pain related to inflamed plantar fascia

Anatomy:
- Plantar fascia originates at the anterior plantar calcaneus and fans out at the distal aspect of the medial longitudinal arch to insert on the metatarsals

Procedure:
- Medial approach is significantly less painful than plantar approach
- Prep skin sterilely. Patient actively dorsiflexes foot and great toe, which will accentuate medial margin of the plantar fascia. Palpate the anterior calcaneus and insert a 1½ in. 25-gauge needle superior to the plantar fascia. Spread the solution in a fan pattern at the origin of the fascia (Figure 2.8)

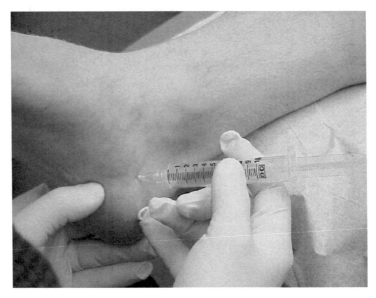

**Figure 2.8.** Plantar fascia injection

**Medication:**
- 1–2 cc betamethasone (Celestone 6 mg/cc) in 3 cc lidocaine (1%)
- 1–2 cc triamcinolone (40 mg/cc) in 3 cc lidocaine (1%)

**Precautions:**
- Avoid injection into the calcaneal fat pad, which can cause fat atrophy
- Avoid injection into the medial plantar nerve

# 3 Environmental Injuries

## High Altitude Injuries

### 3.1 ACUTE MOUNTAIN SICKNESS (AMS)

Br J Sports Med 1999;33:376; Mayo Clin Proc 1998;73:988
**Cause:**
  • Hypoxia associated with rapid ascent to altitude
**Epidem:**
  • Altitude illness develops at elevations above 2000–2400 m, the elevation of most ski resorts in the western United States
  • Of low-land residents visiting these altitudes, approximately 25% develop acute mountain sickness
  • Up to 54% of people traveling abruptly to altitudes above 4000 m develop AMS
  • 20% of experienced climbers develop symptoms of AMS
  • Others at risk include balloon riders, campers, and passengers in unpressurized aircraft (e.g., parachutists)
  • Children more susceptible than adults
  • Alcohol consumption, smoking, and rigorous exercise upon arrival to altitude predispose to AMS
**Pathophys:**
  • Oxygen saturation drops below 90% at 2500 m in most people
  • Hypoxia leads to low arterial oxygenation in cerebral blood flow, which leads to hyperventilation and respiratory alkalosis
  • Sodium retention resulting from hypoxia to the sodium pump leads to fluid retention
  • Rapid ascent does not allow the body to acclimate to these changes

**Sx:**
- Throbbing headache, malaise, lethargy, anorexia, sleep disturbances, nausea, vomiting, and a dry cough or mild dyspnea
- Typically develop within 8–24 hours of ascent and resolve without specific treatment in 24–72 hours

**Si:**
- Tachycardia
- Peripheral fluid retention (edema)

**Crs:**
- Generally benign, self-limited condition that resolves without sequellae
- Failure to improve within 24–48 hours and/or the development of pulmonary or neurologic symptoms may indicate the development of high-altitude cerebral edema (HACE) or high-altitude pulmonary edema (HAPE)

**Cmplc:** High-altitude cerebral edema (see 3.2)
High-altitude pulmonary edema (see 3.2)
Respiratory failure and death

**DiffDx:** Acute MI, CHF, pulmonary embolism (PE), caffeine or sympathomimetic ingestion, anemia, pneumonia

**Lab:**
- None; however, other causes of AMS symptoms should be entertained (toxins, hypoglycemia, meningitis, etc.)

**Rx:**
- Stop the ascent and rest or plan acclimatization day in air travel to altitude
- Avoid alcohol and vigorous exercise early at altitude. Moderate exercise assists with acclimatization
- Acetaminophen or ibuprofen may help alleviate the headache
- Antiemetics may help alleviate the nausea
- Acetazolamide (Diamox) 250 mg tid is a carbonic anhydrase inhibitor that stimulates ventilation and can improve the symptoms of AMS; in more severe cases or in those allergic to sulfas, dexamethasone (Decadron) 2–4 mg every 6 hours followed by a taper, may be used
- Descent from altitude, oxygen therapy, and hyperbaric treatment are generally not necessary for AMS

## 3.2 HIGH-ALTITUDE CEREBRAL EDEMA (HACE) AND PULMONARY EDEMA (HAPE)

Med Sci Sports Exerc 1994;26:195; Crit Care Clin 1999;15:265

Cause:
- High-altitude cerebral edema (HACE) is associated with rising intracranial pressure
- High-altitude pulmonary edema (HAPE) is an exaggerated pulmonary hypertension caused by hemodynamic dysfunction from an acute hypoxic state

Epidem:
- Risk factors include: elevation attained, speed of ascent, and a history of previous HAPE. Strenuous exercise performed immediately upon arrival to altitude may also contribute
- The reported incidence ranges from 0.01 to 15.5% of those ascending to high altitude
- Mortality of HACE approaches 60% if coma ensues
- A genetic predisposition may exist

Pathophys:
- The mechanism of injury in HACE is not well-understood, but is probably related to hypoxic cerebral vasodilation
- Sympathetic vasoconstrictor overactivity and endothelial dysfunction (impaired nitric oxide release and augmented endothelin-1 release) may contribute to pulmonary hypertension in HAPE-prone individuals
    - Hypoxic pulmonary vasoconstriction leads to hyperperfusion and alveolar flooding
    - The discrepancy between perfusion and ventilation in portions of the lung is the most likely pathophysiology in HAPE
    - Other mechanisms may also contribute to HAPE including sympathetic nervous system discharge from cerebral vasodilation

Sx:
- Symptoms of AMS are present with all forms of altitude injury and include headache, nausea, vomiting, anorexia, lightheadedness, dizziness, and are worsened by exertion
- Typical symptoms of HACE include unrelenting headache associated with vomiting, truncal ataxia, impaired mental status (confusion, poor judgment, delirium), and severe lassitude

ENVIRONMENTAL INJURIES

Hemiparesis, hemiplegia, seizures, and coma are less common but suggest progression of this syndrome. HACE can develop within 24 hours of AMS but typically will be delayed 1 to 3 days

- HAPE symptoms are mostly respiratory and include dyspnea, cough, fatigue, chest pain, weakness, and lethargy. Cough may be frothy or blood-stained as a result of capillary distension and leakage

**Si:**

- Patients developing HACE may show nonspecific neurologic deficits (ranging from ataxia to coma) in addition to the signs of AMS (tachycardia, generalized edema)
- HAPE patients can show tachypnea, orthopnea, tachycardia, low grade fever and cyanosis
- Lung auscultation may reveal rales, but the degree of crackles may not reflect the severity of pulmonary compromise

**Crs:**

- Although AMS is a generally benign, self-limiting condition that improves with acclimation, HACE and HAPE are very dangerous clinical syndromes requiring prompt treatment as pulmonary failure and death may occur with hours of symptom onset
- Symptoms of HACE or HAPE can resolve within a few days if immediate descent and treatment have occurred
- Previous episodes increase the risk for future recurrence
- Prevention is important
    Ascend no more than 2000 m per day
    Maximize physical conditioning and climbing experience before entering high altitude environments
    Avoid dehydration, medications, alcohol, and tobacco

**Cmplc:** Respiratory failure and death

**DiffDx:** Acute MI, CHF, PE, severe anemia, drug overdose (caffeine or sympathomimetic), pneumonia

**Lab:**

- Arterial blood gas (if available) may demonstrate hypoxia and may be useful to show improvement with therapy
- Other causes of altered mental status and cardiopulmonary disease should be ruled out with any means necessary (chemistry, CSF, CBC)

**Xray:**

- Chest radiograph may be normal or appear as mild congestive heart failure

**Rx:**
- Descent from altitude is key
- Oxygen (2–4 L/min)
- Dexamethasone (Decadron) 4–8 mg IV q4 hours may be helpful in HACE, especially when descent is delayed
- Nifedipine 10 mg tid (Procardia), hydralazine 10–25 mg qid (Apresoline), phentolamine 5–10 mg in 10 mL NS local injection (Regitine) and nitric oxide have been shown to improve HAPE experimentally by lowering pulmonary artery pressure
- Diuretics, morphine, steroids, and antibiotics have not been shown to improve the symptoms or outcome of HAPE
- Hyperbaric treatment, if available, is recommended to improve arterial oxygenation and limit the cascade of events that lead to irreparable HACE and/or HAPE

# Cold Weather Injuries

## 3.3 NON-FREEZING INJURIES: TRENCH FOOT (IMMERSION FOOT)

Arch Intern Med 1991;151:785

**Cause:**
- Prolonged exposure of feet to cold in wet footwear

**Epidem:**
- More common in temperatures 32–50°F

**Pathophys:**
- No actual freezing of tissue, but injury results from prolonged cooling
- Three stages of injury: ischemic (hours to days); hyperemic (days to weeks); recovery (weeks to months)

**Sx:**
- *Ischemic phase*—cold, tingling followed by numbness, worsening pain, and inability to move foot
- *Hyperemic phase*—severe burning pain and reappearance of proximal sensation

- *Recovery phase*—hypersensitivity to cold may persist long-term; severe cases may lead to permanent disability

**Si:**
- *Ischemic phase*—pale mottled skin, pulses and sensation are decreased or absent
- *Hyperemic phase*—edema, blisters, ulcers, tissue sloughing, and gangrene are possible
- *Recovery phase*—hyperhidrosis and cold hypersensitivity may persist long-term

**Crs:**
- Usually complete resolution if treated early
- Duration of exposure and degree of area involved correlates to length of healing

**Cmplc:** Cellulitis; ischemia

**DiffDx:** Ischemic limb

**Rx:**
- Treatment is supportive
- Gentle warming and drying of affected skin
- Elevation and soft, clean dry dressings
- Check for updated tetanus status
- Wear soft, loose footwear and limit strenuous activities

## 3.4 NON-FREEZING INJURIES: CHILBLAINS (PERNIO)

Clin Sports Med 1989;8:111

**Cause:**
- Exposure to cold air or moisture for prolonged period of time

**Epidem:**
- More common in women and children
- Raynaud's disease can predispose to chilblains

**Pathophys:**
- Abnormal peripheral vasoconstrictive response

**Sx:**
- Cold, numbness, pain, and pruritis in affected area, usually the extremities or face

**Si:**
- Cutaneous manifestations occur up to 12 hours after exposure
- Initially—localized erythema, cyanosis, nodules, affecting mostly lower extremities, toes, hands, and ears
- Later—ulceration, vesicles, and bullae

**Crs:**
- Usually complete resolution if treated early
- Length of exposure correlated to length of healing
- Affected areas are more prone to reinjury

**Cmplc:** Cellulitis

**DiffDx:** Raynaud's disease, ischemic limb

**Rx:**
- Upon rewarming there may be intense pruritus, burning parasthesias, and tender blue nodules that can persist for 14 days
- Treatment is mainly supportive
- Nifedipine (Procardia) 20 mg tid has been shown to have prophylactic and therapeutic benefit
- Topical corticosteroids or a brief oral steroid burst may be beneficial

## 3.5 NON-FREEZING INJURIES: COLD URTICARIA

J Am Acad Dermatol 1992;26:306

**Cause:**
- Cold-induced mast cell-mediated generalized urticarial reaction

**Epidem:**
- No age or sex predilection

**Pathophys:**
- IgG-mediated allergic hypersensitivity

**Sx:**
- Fatigue, headache, dyspnea, tachycardia
- Rarely, anaphylactic shock

**Si:**
- Local or generalized wheals, edema, and erythema

**Crs:**
- Recovery is complete, however, individuals may become sensitized and be at higher risk at higher temperatures later on

**Cmplc:** Cellulitis

**DiffDx:** Drug induced urticaria, exercise induced urticaria (see 23.5), cholinergic urticaria (see 23.6)

**Lab:**
- Cryoglobulins, cryofibrinogens, cold agglutinins, or hemolysins may be present in a minority of patients

**Other Testing:**
- *Ice water immersion test*—immersion of an extremity in an ice bath precipitates angioedema of the distal portion with urticaria at air interface within minutes of the challenge

**Rx:**
- Minimize cold exposure—the rate of cooling is more important than the absolute temperature achieved
- Periactin, doxepin or hydroxyzine for acute pruritis or urticaria, if severe
- Fexofenadine (Allegra) 60 mg daily, loratadine (Claritin) 10 mg daily, or cetirizine (Zyrtec) 5 mg daily may be beneficial for prophylaxis

## 3.6 FREEZING INJURIES: FROSTBITE

J Trauma 2000;48:171

**Cause:**
- Exposure to freezing elements

**Epidem:**
- More common in the winter and at higher altitudes
- Poor acclimation and failure to anticipate potential for extreme exposures are risk factors affecting outdoor enthusiasts

**Pathophys:**
- Intense vasoconstriction occurs as part of the body's temperature-conserving reaction
- Frostnip is the initial superficial vasoconstrictive response that can lead to frostbite the longer and more extreme the exposure occurs
- Frostbite is characterized microscopically as reversible ice crystal formation in the intracellular and extracellular spaces, along with hyperosmolar changes and intracellular damage
- Three degrees of frostbite are differentiated by the degrees of tissue damage that occur during the rewarming phases

1. *First degree*: injury to superficial skin layers
2. *Second degree*: injury extends to dermis and subdermis fat cells
3. *Third degree*: injury to deeper tissues including muscle tendon, bone

**Sx:**

- Initially, all degrees present similarly with coldness, pain, numbness, and redness
- Exposed skin is at highest risk, such as the face, ears, fingers
- Later symptoms may only be anesthesia and paralysis of the affected area

**Si:**

- Early on, signs indicating the degree of frostbite may not be known until the thawing period has begun
- *Frostnip*—digits become hyperemic after thawing, with associated paresthesia, but no evidence of tissue damage or edema
- *First-degree*—thawing is painful and associated with erythema and edema; skin can become waxy in texture at this stage
- *Second-degree*—erythema and edema progress into vesicles and straw-colored blisters
- *Third-degree*—pain is less severe or nonexistent; blisters may be filled with serosanguinous fluid or frank blood

**Crs:**

- Signs of favorable recovery: rapid return to normal temperature, return of sensation, clear blisters, brisk capillary refill time distally, pink skin that blanches
- Signs of poor recovery: cold, blue tissue without blisters, hard, white insensitive skin; dark red or blue tissue that does not blanch; absence of edema; superimposed trauma; signs of tissue necrosis; and history of freeze–thaw–refreeze
- Duration of exposure and degree of area involved correlates to length of healing
- May be hypersensitive to cold weather; long-term extra protection against cold exposure and immersion necessary

**Cmplc:** Chronic pain, limb or digital ischemia and necrosis, cellulitis

**DiffDx:** Peripheral vascular embolic ischemia, deep vein thrombosis (DVT)

**Lab:**

- In more severe cases, initial and serial laboratory studies include CBC, serum electrolytes, Ca, albumin, amylase, creatine kinase, LFTs, coagulation studies, and UA

**Other Testing:**
- Core temperature monitoring
- ECG, chest radiograph
- Patients with severe electrolyte disturbances may require telemetry during initial phase of admission

**Rx:**
- Frostnip is best treated with gentle rewarming
- Other degrees of frostbite require more significant measures:
  Rapid warming in 45°C water bath
  Handling and drying of affected skin should be gentle; no massaging of affected areas
  Pain medication
  Warmed (37°C) intravenous fluids
  Avoid ointments, alcohol, tobacco
  Elevation of extremities and application of soft, clean dry dressings
  Leave blisters alone; broken blisters should be cleaned thoroughly and aloe vera applied
  Antibiotics not necessary for minor injury, but penicillin should be considered in a field setting
  Tetanus booster should be given
- Special considerations for advanced-degree frostbite:
  Referral for sympathectomy, either medical or surgical
  Occupational therapy rehabilitation
  Amputation in most severe cases

## 3.7 HYPOTHERMIA

Med Clin N Amer 1994;78:305; Surg Clin North Amer 1995;75:243; Ann Emerg Med 1993;22:370

**Cause:**
- Requires two factors: the ambient temperature must be below core body temperature (CBT) and the body's ability to generate heat must be less than ongoing heat losses

**Epidem:**
- Hypothermia occurs commonly in water sports (boating, swimming, scuba, white water rafting), winter sports, and mountaineering

- It is also quite common in endurance events where the exhausted participant is unable to maintain heat production to overcome environmental losses
- Major risk factors divided into two categories, those which result in greater heat losses (through impaired thermoregulation) and those leading to reduced thermogenesis. These include age (the very old and young), underlying diseases (cardiovascular, endocrinopathies), exhaustive exercise, alcohol intoxication, and trauma

**Pathophys:**
- Heat produced by basal metabolism is adequate to maintain CBT at 37°C with ambient air temperatures above 28°C (82.4°F). Exercise produces heat allowing thermostasis at lower ambient temperatures
- Certain environmental conditions can also overwhelm the thermogenic potential, as is seen in cold water immersion or extreme windchill
- Heat loss occurs through four transfer processes: conduction, convection, evaporation, and radiation
- Hypothermia is defined as a CBT below 35°C and is further divided into mild (CBT 32–35°C), moderate (CBT 28–32°C), and severe (CBT <28°C)
- Cold effects the function of multiple body systems including the cardiovascular, pulmonary, urinary, hemocoagulation, and central nervous systems

**Si/Sx:**
- Mild hypothermia characterized by tachycardia, uncontrolled shivering, and peripheral vasoconstriction. Cold diuresis, common in the early stages of hypothermia, occurs in response to the increasing central blood pool caused by peripheral vasoconstriction
- Other findings in mild hypothermia including dysarthria, extremity ataxia, skin pallor, perioral cyanosis, and muscle rigidity. Deep tendon reflexes are initially brisk but will diminish as cooling continues
- With CBT below 32°C, the body's ability to respond becomes significantly impaired. The shivering reflex is lost and heat production falls sharply. Hypotension and bradycardia are common, with a 50% reduction in heart rate, at temperatures below 25°C
- Worsening cognitive function can contribute further by preventing the victims from recognizing their danger and seeking warmth
- Reduced cerebral blood flow leads to obtundation, stupor, and coma. Pupillary dilation, muscular rigidity, loss of reflexes, and

unresponsiveness may lead to the mistaken conclusion that the victim is dead
- Cardiac arrhythmias become common at CBT below 32°C. Atrial fibrillation frequently occurs in the moderate hypothermic range and is probably due to atrial distention. Supraventricular tachycardia is also common, particularly during rewarming. As the temperature falls below 28°C, ventricular irritability leads to more severe arrhythmias including ventricular tachycardia and fibrillation. Spontaneous asystole or fine ventricular fibrillation occurs at temperatures below 20–25°C

**Lab:**
- Bleeding time increased
- BUN increases

**ECG:**
- ECG changes associated with hypothermia include the arrythmias described previously
- The Osborne wave ("J" wave) forms at the junction of the QRS complex and T wave giving the ST segment a characteristic J shape. It is typically seen at temperatures below 32°C in leads II and V$_6$. As temperature falls, it becomes prominent in leads V$_3$ and V$_4$. It is reported in approximately 80% of patients with a CBT below 30°C

**Crs:**
- Aggressive monitoring and fluid replacement are required during rewarming to avoid serious hypovolemic complications
- One potentially fatal complication during rewarming is CBT afterdrop. Afterdrop refers to the continued core cooling during early rewarming. Two factors contribute to this phenomenon
    Equilibration of blood temperature as the cold blood from the extremities is mobilized and mixes with the central pool (conductive loss)
    The cooling of warm blood from the central pool as it perfuses the cold peripheral tissues (convective loss); the temperature drop due to this phenomenon can be significant and may lead to a worsening condition in the face of aggressive rewarming

**Cmplc:** Frostbite (see 3.6), disseminated intravascular coagulation (DIC), cerebral vascular accident (CVA), refractory ventricular fibrillation, failure to warm prior to cessation of resuscitative efforts

**DiffDx:** Rigor mortis (death)

**Rx:**

- Early recognition and prompt rewarming are critical
- Full recovery, even from extremely low temperature may be possible and full resuscitative efforts should be undertaken even in the severely hypothermic patient
- Active external rewarming techniques (chemical hot packs, warming blankets or pads, and radiant heat lamps) are usually adequate to warm the mildly hypothermic patient and result in a warming rate of approximately 0.5–1°C per hour
- Internal rewarming refers to the introduction of heat directly to the victim's core

  Heated inhalation therapy: use of heated humidified air or oxygen (42–46°C) delivered through endotracheal tube or mask

  IV hydration (isotonic crystalloid solution 5% glucose warmed to 40–42°C) has dual indication in the hypothermic patient both as a rewarming technique and to provide intravascular volume replacement

  Peritoneal lavage: following the percutaneous placement of an 8 F catheter into the pelvic gutter, warmed isotonic dialysate (40–45°C) is introduced in allocates of 1 to 2 L. This fluid is aspirated after 20–30 mins. A 6-L per h exchange rate (10–20 cc/kg) results in rewarming at 1–3°C per hour

  Extracorporeal rewarming (ECR): this very effective method uses cardiopulmonary bypass equipment for rewarming in the severely hypothermic patients. Advantages with ECR include the ability to control the rate of rewarming and continue tissue perfusion and oxygenation in the setting of cardiac arrest

- The patient should be handled very gently with continuous cardiac monitoring as well as close attention to blood pressure. The accurate assessment of the CBT is also crucial. A rectal or esophageal thermistor, placed 15–20 cm into the lumen of the viscera, provides an efficient means for continuous CBT monitoring
- Arrhythmias: the predominant atrial arrhythmia associated with hypothermia is fibrillation with a slow ventricular response. Atrial fibrillation usually resolves with rewarming and does not require specific therapy. Supraventricular tachyarrythmias are common during rewarming, but these also resolve as the CBT rises. The calcium channel blockers typically used to treat supraventricular tachyarrythmias are not effective at low temperatures. Ventricular arrhythmias tend to be resistant to treatment as long as the patient

remains cold. At temperatures below 30°C, bretylium is the most useful antiarrhythmic
- The decision to stop resuscitative efforts is a complex one. The statement "a patient isn't dead until they are warm and dead" has shown merit many times in the past with heroic saves of profoundly hypothermic victims

# Heat Injuries

## 3.8 HYPERTHERMIA

Crit Care Clin 1999;15:251

**Cause:**
- Failure of body's ability to thermoregulate in the face of elevated environmental temperature, extreme physical exertion, and/or disease state affecting the body's ability to effectively dissipate heat

**Epidem:**
- More common in the summer and in warm climates
- Poor acclimation and failure to anticipate potential for extreme exposures are risk factors affecting outdoor enthusiasts
- Elderly people, those taking vasoconstrictive drugs, smokers, and extreme athletes are at higher risk
- Mortality from heat stroke is 10%, usually due to arrhythmia, shock, cardiac ischemia, or renal dysfunction

**Pathophys:**
- Inability of the body to effectively thermoregulate causes elevated temperature
- Evaporative losses worsen dehydration and subsequent sodium loss
- Electrolyte disturbances lead to muscle breakdown and rhabdomyolysis, which can lead to renal failure
- The spectrum of heat injury is differentiated by the degrees of systemic changes that develop
  - *Heat syncope*—loss of consciousness characterized by cutaneous vasodilation with consequent systemic and cerebral hypotension
  - *Heat cramps*—muscular cramps caused by electrolyte and fluid depletion

     *Heat exhaustion*—fatigue, weakness, and other systemic symptoms
       resulting from prolonged heat exposure, dehydration, and
       electrolyte depletion
     *Heat stroke*—life-threatening cerebral dysfunction resulting from a
       failure of the thermoregulatory mechanism

**Sx:**

- Symptoms of heat injuries are common to all categories and grow
  worse as duration of exposure and delay of treatment increase
  *Heat syncope*—fatigue, thirst, lightheadedness, and headache
  *Heat cramps*—muscular cramps, pain, and spasms
  *Heat exhaustion*—fatigue, weakness, anxiety, impaired judgement,
     hyperventilation, and other systemic symptoms
  *Heat stroke*—impaired consciousness, nausea, and seizures

**Si:**

- Absence of sweating reflects advanced injury and the highest risk for
  heat stroke
- Symptoms of heat injuries progress from mild discomfort to
  systemic compromise with increasing temperature
  *Heat syncope*—rapid pulse and hypotension
  *Heat cramps*—skin moist and cool, profuse sweating, palpable
     muscle twitching, normal to slightly elevated core temperature
  *Heat exhaustion*—core temperature >37.8°C, rapid pulse, mental
     status changes
  *Heat stroke*—high fever (>41°C), seizure activity, delirium,
     rhabdomyolysis

**Crs:**

- Signs of favorable recovery: rapid return to normal temperature,
  maintenance of isotonic volume, lack of central nervous systemic
  symptoms
- Signs of poor recovery: delayed removal from hot environment,
  prolonged dehydration, electrolyte disturbance, coexisting morbidity
  (age, heart disease, obesity, trauma)
- Exertional heat injury, such as that experienced by marathon
  runners and triathletes, carries a more favorable prognosis
- Previous heat injury is a risk for subsequent injury and should be
  considered in risk prevention

**Cmplc:** Disseminated intravascular coagulation (DIC)
       Rhabdomyolysis (see 22.2)
       Death

**ENVIRONMENTAL INJURIES**

**DiffDx:** Malignant hyperthermia, neuroleptic malignant syndrome (NMS), febrile illness (see 22.1, 22.2)

**Lab:**
- Initial tests—UA to demonstrate ketonuria and early dehydration, renal function tests and serum sodium
- Later tests—serial UA, urine myoglobin, serum chemistries to include potassium, phosphorus and calcium, creatine kinase, CBC
- Consider blood alcohol level and screening for illicit substances

**Other Testing:**
- Core temperature monitoring
- ECG—ST changes suggesting ischemia, peaked T waves of hyperkalemia
- Patients with severe electrolyte disturbances may require telemetry during initial hospitalization

**Rx:**
- Heat syncope is treated with rest, sitting in a cool place, and oral fluid rehydration
- Heat cramps are treated as above, but intravenous fluids may be necessary to deliver sufficient isotonic saline more rapidly; sodium tablets are not recommended because of their slow absorption
- Heat exhaustion is treated as above, but also includes more aggressive initial intravenous fluid replacement (1–2 L over 2–4 h) and more prolonged therapy (up to 24 h); IV 3% (hypertonic) saline may be necessary if sodium depletion is severe
- There are three major considerations for treating heat stroke
    1. Initially, rapid cooling to bring the core temperature to below 39°C, using ice baths, fans, and cold compresses. Gastric lavage and submersion are minimally effective, but not recommended because of practicality and interference with monitoring. Antipyretics are not effective for environmentally induced hyperthermia and are contraindicated. Anti-seizure medications are probably not necessary until the core temperature is reduced (chlorpromazine 25–50 mg or diazepam 5–10 mg IV can be helpful in this regard).
    2. Management of shock—both hypovolemic and/or cardiogenic—is critical. Central venous pressure monitoring may be necessary to allow rapid, aggressive volume replacement without overloading the circulation.
    3. Close monitoring for systemic complications such as rhabdomyolysis, renal failure, DIC, cardiac arrhythmias, and

serious electrolyte disturbances is key. Fluid administration should be sufficient to maintain high urine output (>50 mL/h). Use of mannitol (0.25 mg/kg) and alkalinizing the urine (IV sodium bicarbonate, 250 mL of 4%) should be considered.

# 4 Nutrition and Ergogenics

Nutrition guidelines are established every 5 years by the U.S. Department of Agriculture and the U.S. Department of Health and Human Services (http://www.nalusda.gov/fnic/dga/dguide95.html). The Food Guide Pyramid (http://www.nal.usda.gov:8001/py/pmap.htm) offers the average American a general guide for a healthy diet.

## BANNED DRUGS

For the most current list of drugs banned by the National Collegiate Athletic Association (NCAA) and the International Olympic Committee, check the websites listed below.
- <http://www.ncaa.org/sports_sciences/drugtesting/banned_list.html>
- <http://www.olympic.org/ioc/e/org/medcom/medcom_antidopage _e.html>

---

**Table 4.1. Nutrition Guide for Optimum Performance**

Eat a high carbohydrate diet.
Taper by decreasing the intensity and/or duration of practice for 1–2 days before competition.
Eat a carbohydrate meal 3–4 hours before competition.
Maintain adequate fluid intake before and during competition.
Avoid sugar less than 1 hour before competition.
After exhausting exercise, eat carbohydrates.
Eat foods containing adequate vitamins and minerals.

---

## 4.1 CREATINE

Clin Sport Med 1999;18:651; Nut Aspects of Ex 1999;18:651; Phy Sportmed 1999;27(5):47

**Cause:** Oral supplementation

**Pathophys:**
- Short burst intense exercise rapidly consumes ATP
- Phosphocreatine serves as an energy buffer transferring its phosphate group to ADP to regenerate ATP
- There is four to six times more creatine phosphate (CP) than ATP stored in cells
- Both of these energy sources are depleted within 6–10 sec of intensive exercise, and they are replenished primarily through breakdown of carbohydrates and fats
- Ergogenic effects
    - Creatine stores in muscle are increased through the ingestion of creatine (at most about 20%)
    - Increasing the supply of creatine phosphate provides more energy to exercising muscle
    - Creatine improves performance in short-duration, repetitive, and intense exercise; improvement in cycling, swimming, kayaking, rowing, weight lifting, jumping, and sprinting ability has been shown
    - Creatine increases total body mass and fat-free muscle mass (0.5–2.0 kg)
    - Creatine decreases lactic acid levels in the blood during sprints
    - Conversely, creatine does not improve isometric strength, power, or aerobic endurance
    - Middle-aged athletes may benefit more than younger athletes
    - Men seem to benefit more than women from creatine use
    - Simultaneous training exercise is required for a beneficial effect
    - Creatine use with exercise results in increases in muscle mass; type I (slow twitch, aerobic), type IIA (intermediate, anaerobic), and type IIB (fast twitch, anaerobic) muscle mass is increased
    - Caffeine reduces the efficacy of creatine
    - Large carbohydrate intake augments muscle uptake of creatine

**Sx:** Muscle cramps (25% of users), strains, decreased urine output, diarrhea

**Cmplc:** There are some reports of association with exertional rhabdomyolysis and heat injuries probably related to poor hydration, cardiac arrhythmia, cardiomyopathy, DVT, seizure, and use of other ergogenic substances

**Lab:** UA, BUN/Cr, or other labs indicated by presentation

**Rx:**
- A loading dose of 0.3 g per kg of body weight per day (0.14 g per lb of body weight per d) divided over 4–5 doses per day is taken for 5–7 days
- A maintenance dose of 0.03 g per kg of body weight per day (0.014 g per lb of body weight per d) is subsequently taken
- Naturally available creatine is found in beef, dairy products, and fish
- Not recommended for adolescents

## 4.2 ANABOLIC STEROIDS

Clin Sport Med 1999;18:667; Am J Sport Med 1993;21:468

**Cause:** Oral or injectable supplementation

**Epidem:** 6.6% of high school male seniors; also used by the recreational athlete looking for rapid gains

**Pathophys:**
- Testosterone is produced in the testes and adrenals
- Androstenedione is produced in the adrenal gland and testes then converted in the liver to testosterone
- Testosterone affects almost all body tissues by decreasing tissue breakdown and increasing tissue production
- Excess testosterone is peripherally converted to estrogen resulting in feminization in males (Ann Pharm 1992;26:520)
- Size and strength gains through anticatabolic, anabolic, and motivational effects

    Anticatabolic—displacement of cortisol from receptors resulting in less wasting and negative nitrogen balance

    Anabolic effect—induce protein synthesis, stimulation of endogenous HGH

    Motivational—aggressiveness to train hard
- Effects are reversed as soon as the steroids are stopped

**Sx:** Significant improvement in performance more than indicated by level of training; muscle hypertrophy; aggressiveness and mood swings; risk taking behaviors; premature cardiovascular disease

**Si:** Muscular hypertrophy; acne; striae; elevated BP; gynectomastia; gonadal atrophy and impaired spermatogenesis, clitorimegaly, male pattern baldness

**Cmplc:** Sudden death, myocardial infarction, increased low-density lipoproteins (LDL), decreased high-density lipoproteins (HDL), hypertension, concentric cardiac hypertrophy, hypercoagulability, decreased spermatogenesis, decreased testicle size, prostate hypertrophy, prostate cancer, voice alterations, liver damage and cancer, premature epiphyseal closure with resulting short stature, weaker tendons (Achilles and patellar tendon rupture), electrolyte imbalances, insulin resistance, skin pathology, aggression, depression, and paranoia, HIV and Hep B and C

**Lab:** Sperm count, electrolytes, glucose, serum lipids, coagulation studies, liver function tests, PSA (over 40 or 50 years of age), an ECG, and possibly an echocardiogram if indications of ventricular hypertrophy are present; screening for hepatitis B, hepatitis C, and HIV is recommended for any athlete using injectable drugs

**Rx:**
- Stop supplementation
- Management of post-steroid depressive sx and dependence sx
- Multidisciplinary management approach

---

## 4.3 HUMAN GROWTH HORMONE

J Clin Endo and Met 1999;84:3591; Am J Sport Med 1993;21:468
**Cause:** Supplementation by injection
**Epidem:** Unknown
**Pathophys:**
- Growth hormone (somatotropin) is produced in the anterior pituitary gland
- The level of growth hormone increases with exercise and hypoglycemia
- This increase may not occur in obese athletes ( J Clin Endo and Met 1999;84(9):3156)

- Growth hormone increases liver and osteoblast production of insulin-like growth factor (ILGF-I) that has anabolic properties
- Ergogenic effects

    Growth hormone inhibits glucose breakdown and increases the level of free fatty acids that can be used for energy

    Growth hormone increases muscle mass, strength, and endurance

    Growth hormone decreases body fat

    Growth hormone may also increase cardiac output and sweating to help in cooling

**Sx:** Signs of acromegaly (increased skull size with prominent cheek bones, protruding jaw and frontal bossing, spade-like hands)

**Si:** Suggestions include monitoring pulse, blood pressure, heart sounds and size for heart failure, lung sounds for pulmonary edema, joints for arthritis, lymph glands, face and extremities for swelling, hair loss, weight, eye examination for papilledema, prostate mass (digital rectal examination)

**Cmplc:**

- Acromegaly, prostate cancer (Science 1998;279:563), hypertension, heart failure, and arthritis
- Although not well studied, short-term use of growth hormone may result in sodium and fluid retention, flushing, or a feeling of heaviness in the legs
- Osteoporosis, impotence/amenorrhea, myopathy, hypertension, diabetes, peripheral neuropathy
- HIV, Hep B and C
- Significant cost (up to $30,000/yr)

**Lab:**

- PSA (over 40 or 50 years of age), bone age for premature closure of epiphyses, glucose, and serum lipids; monitoring for hepatitis B, hepatitis C, and HIV is indicated in athletes using needles for administration
- Current assays to detect abuse of recombinant human growth hormone are of insufficient sensitivity and specificity to prove useful, especially in light of the large fluctuations that may be greater than 100-fold in athletes
- Collagen and procollagen markers are being studied as possible tests for abuse

**Rx:** Stop supplementation and screen for complications

## 4.4 ERYTHROPOIETIN (EPO AND rEPO)

Am J Sport Med 1996;24:PS004
**Cause:** IV or SQ supplementation
**Epidem:** Increased use with availability of rEPO
**Pathophys:**

- EPO is manufactured through an enzyme produced in adult kidneys and fetal livers
- Erythropoietin is produced in response to hypoxia, and it stimulates bone marrow production of erythrocytes
- A synthetic recombinant erythropoietin (rEPO) is available
- Ergogenic effects
    Erythropoietin use results in higher hematocrit, muscle glycogen, and free fatty acids
    After endurance exercise, lactic acid levels are lower
    Erythropoietin used in athletes for 6 weeks was shown to increase maximal oxygen consumption ($Vo_2$ max) and endurance
    Before the advent of rEPO, transfusion with 1–2 L of blood also resulted in increased maximal oxygen uptake and performance

**Sx:** Headache, sx of DVT/PE, exertional collapse
**Si:** Hypertension, signs of DVT/PE
**Cmplc:** Myalgia, hyperviscosity, hypercoagulability, hypertension, and dehydration; DVT, PE, CVA, sudden death
**DiffDx:** Blood doping or altitude training effect; polycythemia vera
**Lab:** Suggested monitoring should include hemoglobin and hematocrit at minimum; other laboratory studies for hepatitis B, hepatitis C, and HIV should be included for athletes using intravenous medications
**Rx:** Stop the supplementation and monitor for complications

## 4.5 STIMULANTS

Clin Sport Med 1997;16:375; The Hughston Clinic Sports Medicine Book, Williams & Wilkins, Baltimore, 1995
**Cause:** Oral supplementation or ingestion of caffeine, amphetamines, dietary or decongestant OTC meds (phenylpropanolamine, pseudophedrine, ephedrine), or other supplements; "Ripped Fuel,"

"Bishops, Brigham, and Mormon Teas," and other herbals containing *ma huang*

**Epidem:** Widespread use in all sports (esp. caffeine)

**Pathophys:**
- Stimulants enhance mental alertness and possess sympathomimetic effects
- Stimulants increase pulse, blood pressure, cardiac output, heart rate, respiratory rate, metabolic rate, and serum glucose
- Ergogenic effects
    More recent studies of amphetamines show no increased performance in sprint and middle distance running, sprint and middle distance swimming, combination cycling and running endurance, endurance while bench stepping with weights, or reaction time
    Some very early studies showed possible benefit in swimming, throwing, shot put, and endurance without increase in speed
    Caffeine, on the other hand, improved endurance cycling performance by 19.5%
    Fat use increased, and carbohydrate use decreased
    Nicotine in smokeless tobacco may decrease strength and power

**Sx:**
- Aerobic exercise intolerance (rapid rise in HR)
- Amphetamines may cause palpitations, psychosis, restlessness, dizziness, insomnia, motor tics, dry mouth, diarrhea or constipation, anorexia, impotence, or change in libido
- Cocaine causes excitement, restlessness, anxiety, confusion, increased sympathetic tone, nausea, vomiting, abdominal pain, seizures, elevated body temperature, chills, and unconsciousness
- Caffeine may cause headache, excitement, agitation, tinnitus, tremors, palpitations, and even seizures
- Sympathomimetics may cause anxiety, agitation, paranoia, hypertension, and palpitations

**Si:** Hypertension, tachycardia, arrhythmia, mental confusion, tremor

**Cmplc:** Arrhythmia with complication, MI, seizure, CVA/TIA, sudden death, weight loss

**DiffDx:** Pheochromocytoma, anxiety state

**Lab:** Urine vanillylmandelic acid (VMA), metanephrines, and 5-hydroxyindoleacetic acid (5-HIAA) levels may be increased with caffeine use, leading to a misdiagnosis of pheochromocytoma; EKG to eval rhythm

**Rx:**

- Caffeine is probably ergogenic between 250–350 mg, which is found in approximately 1–2 cups of regular coffee or 5–7 cans of caffeinated soda taken 1 hour before exercise. The maximum safe dosage of caffeine even for emergency indications is approximately 500 mg per dose or 2500 mg per day
- Stop/withhold other stimulants when more symptomatic

# Section II

# ORTHOPEDIC PROBLEMS

# 5 Cervical Spine Injuries

## 5.1 CERVICAL STRAIN/SPRAIN

**(Ligamentous Sprain, Neck Strain, Whiplash, Myofascial Neck Pain)**
Phy Sportsmed 1997;25:60

**Cause:** Strain is injury to muscle-tendon unit; sprain is ligamentous or capsular injury

**Epidem:** The most common athletic cervical spine injuries; often due to rapid and excessive range of motion in one or more planes

**Pathophys:** The anterior longitudinal ligament prevents hyperextension. Injury to this ligament results in a "whiplash." The posterior longitudinal ligament prevents hyperflexion. Additional support is provided by the ligamentum flavum, interspinous ligaments, ligamentum nuchae. Soft tissue injury involving these supportive muscles and ligaments of the neck

**Sx:** Nonradicular neck and shoulder pain worsened by motion of neck; decreased cervical range of motion

**Si:** Decreased range of motion in multiple directions; spasm of local musculature may be present; no neurologic dysfunction or bony tenderness

**Crs:** Self-limited; most symptoms resolve completely within 4–6 weeks

**Cmplc:** Cervical spine instability can result if there exists significant ligamentous or capsular disruption; should rule out cervical spine instability if injury is acute. If any neurologic symptoms or decreased cervical range of motion, will require lateral flexion and extension views

**DiffDx:** If acute injury, must rule out cervical spine instability; diagnosis of exclusion, after more serious injuries have been ruled out

**Xray:** If spasm and pain persist after several minutes following injury, radiologic exam should be obtained to rule out more serious injury; radiographs may be normal or show loss of normal lordotic curve

**Rx:** Rest, anti-inflammatory medications, local ice massage, and resting neck in a soft collar; muscle relaxants may be indicated; range of motion rehabilitation incorporating strengthening program

**Return to Activity:** Only when asymptomatic, normal muscle strength, and pain-free full cervical range of motion is present; there should be no neck pain with and without axial compression; no instability noted on radiographs

## 5.2 CERVICAL SPONDYLOSIS/SPINAL STENOSIS

### (Cervical Spine Degenerative Disc Disease, Cervical Spine Degenerative Joint Disease, Osteoarthritis)

Clin Sport Med 1998;17:121; 1990;9:279

**Cause:** Ingrowth of bony spurs or herniation of disc material

**Epidem:** Cervical spine stenosis increases the risk of permanent neurologic injury; highest risk of injury in athletes participating in contact and collision sports

**Pathophys:** Spondylosis is degeneration of intervertebral discs with subsequent osteophytic encroachment. Cervical spinal stenosis is developmental narrowing of the AP diameter of the cervical canal or secondary to spondylosis and degenerative disease. Narrowing (stenosis) of the spinal canal or neural foramen with restriction/compression of the spinal cord. Loss of normal cerebral spinal fluid cushion around the cord or deformation of the cord

**Sx:** Chronic neck pain, stiffness, may complain of radicular pain or myelopathy; may present with intense sharp pain in one or both upper extremities (very similar to "burner" or "stinger")

**Si:** Tenderness to palpation along lateral neck or along the spinous processes; limitations of neck motion, may have radicular symptoms with neck flexion

**Crs:** Depending upon the degree of stenosis, may predispose to spinal cord or nerve root injury, especially with contact/collision sports

**Cmplc:** May develop quadriparesis due to central cord syndrome (contusion of central portion of spinal cord). Transient quadriplegia/cervical cord neuropraxia is an acute transient neurologic episode of cervical cord origin. Findings include both arms, both legs, all 4 extremities, or an ipsilateral arm and leg. Sensory changes are present with or without motor findings. Probability of recurrence depends on spinal canal/vertebral body ratio.

**DiffDx:** Burner/stinger (see 5.4), herniated cervical disc (see 5.3)
**Lab:** If radicular symptoms present, may consider EMG
**Xray:**

- Radiographs, may see sclerosis in the intervertebral disk area with osteophytes; osteophytes may project from the posterior portion of the vertebral body into the spinal canal, causing stenosis; should evaluate Torg (or Pavlov's) ratio of spinal canal diameter to vertebral body diameter; ratio <0.8 implies spinal stenosis
- MRI evaluation of spinal cord diameter to canal diameter is more reliable

**Rx:**

- Rest, nonsteroidal anti-inflammatory medications and observation if symptoms resolving
- Steroids may be indicated (short course, i.e., prednisone 60 mg/d for 5–7 days) for acute pain exacerbations
- Occasional consultation to a pain clinic for epidural steroid injections
- Neurosurgical consult if any complications or recurrent symptoms

**Return to Activity:** Depends on symptomatology and results of radiographic evaluation; generally pain-free ROM, normal strength

## 5.3 CERVICAL RADICULOPATHY

Phys Sportsmed 1997;25:60
**Cause:** Disc protrusion, which may result in nerve root or spinal cord impingement
**Epidem:** Acute injury from compression or hyperflexion injury; chronic due to degeneration of disc
**Pathophys:**

- C2 through C7 are connected in series with intervertebral discs between each vertebral body
- Intervertebral discs are composed of an annulus fibrosus (strong fibrous ring) that surrounds the nucleus pulposus

- Nerve roots exit one each side between the bodies and the transverse processes of adjoining vertebrae (each nerve root exits above the cervical level, i.e. C5 exits between C4 and C5)
- Acute injury due to rupture of the disc where nucleus pulposus extrudes through a tear in the annulus fibrosus
- Chronic symptoms from degeneration of the disc with combination of disc and osteophytic encroachment on the nerve foramen

**Sx:** Neck pain with radiation into shoulder or arm; burning pain, weakness, or sensory changes in the distribution of a specific nerve root; may have upper motor neuron sx in the LE (i.e., bowel or bladder sx)

**Si:** Reproduction of symptoms with compression test or Spurling's maneuver; pain relieved with distraction test; may isolate weakness or neurologic deficits (reflex and/or sensory)
- Compression test
  Examiner applies axial load by applying pressure to the patient's head
  Positive test indicated by reproduction of radicular sx
- Spurling's test (Fig. 5.1)
  Examiner gently extends and laterally flexes the neck
  Positive test indicated by ipsilateral radicular sx
- Distraction test
  Examiner provides axial traction of the c-spine to relieve radicular sx
- Motor function tests

| C1–2 | — | flexion of the head |
| C3 | — | lateral bending of the head |
| C4 | trapezius | shoulder shrug |
| C5 | deltoid | shoulder abduction |
| C5–6 | biceps | elbow flexion |
| C6 | extensor carpi radialis | wrist extension |
| C7 | triceps, finger extensors | elbow extension, finger extension |
| C8 | flexor digitorum | finger flexion |
| C8–T1 | interosseous muscles | finger abduction |

- Dermatome distribution tests

| C2 | upper neck/occiput |
| C3 | lower neck |
| C4 | shoulder tip |
| C5 | lateral arm |

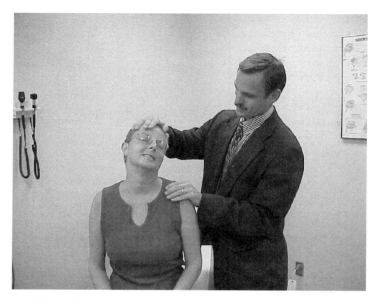

**Figure 5.1.** Spurling's test

| | |
|---|---|
| C6 | lateral forearm and thumb |
| C7 | middle finger |
| C8 | medial forearm and little finger |

- Reflex testing
  | | |
  |---|---|
  | C5–C6 | biceps reflex and brachioradialis reflex |
  | C7–C8 | triceps reflex |

Check LE DTRs

**Crs:** Symptoms usually respond to conservative therapy within 6–12 weeks; if severe neurologic deficits or symptoms persist despite conservative management, surgical consult is warranted

**Cmplc:** Progressive encroachment upon nerve root with escalating symptomatology; association with chronic, recurrent cervical nerve root neuropraxia (burner)

**DiffDx:** Demyelinating conditions, peripheral nerve injury, thoracic outlet syndrome

**Lab:** EMG and NCS to determine nerve root involved and extent

**Xray:**
- Radiographs may show disc space narrowing, anterior bony ridging, and loss of normal cervical lordosis
- CT not very useful in visualizing cervical disc pathology
- MRI to display compression

**Rx:**
- Rest, NSAIDs, muscle relaxants, and/or pain control
- If radicular symptoms present, short course of oral steroids may be indicated (prednisone 60 mg/d for 5–7 days)
- Neck support with soft collar and traction may offer relief
- Gentle active range of motion
- Spinal manipulation should be avoided

**Return to Activity:** Acute injury associated with pain, limited cervical ROM, or neurologic signs or symptoms is an absolute contraindication; chronic degenerative disc disease, if neurologically normal and normal muscle strength and full range of motion is relative contraindication

## 5.4 TRANSIENT BRACHIAL PLEXOPATHY (BURNER, STINGER)

Phys Sportsmed 1996;24:57

**Cause:** Neurologic insult to the brachial plexus or cervical nerve root

**Epidem:** The most common neurologic cervical injury; traction injury to shoulder or compression injury to the neck; common in contact sports such as football and wrestling; most commonly involves C5–C6 nerve distribution

**Pathophys:** A transient, unilateral neuropraxia due to traction of the brachial plexus or compression of the cervical nerve root; more severe lesions may be due to axonotmesis or neurotmesis

**Sx:** Intense sharp, unilateral "burning" paresthesia or weakness in the upper extremity

**Si:** Neurologic dysfunction in sensory and motor may be present but usually resolves within minutes; Spurling's maneuver (see 5.3) positive in compression and negative in traction injury

**Crs:** Initially patients are overtly symptomatic, yet show quick recovery of paresthesia and/or weakness with full range of motion without pain; motor weakness often is not initially apparent and may not appear until several days after the injury; if symptoms do not show evidence of resolution, more severe injury should be sought

**Cmplc:** If symptoms are bilateral or involve the lower extremity, suspect cord neurapraxia, cervical spine fracture, or ligamentous injury

**DiffDx:** Herniated disc (see 5.3) or cervical stenosis (see 5.2)

**Lab:** EMG warranted for persistent symptoms

**Xray:** MRI if persistent neurologic deficit and prolonged or recurrent symptoms

**Rx:**

- First rule out serious cervical spine injury
- Remove from activity until all symptoms resolve
- If injury occurred from axial load injury, first time injury, symptoms persist >15 min, or symptoms are recurrent, imaging studies are warranted to rule out cervical spine stenosis or HNP
- Prevention includes strengthening program for neck and protective neck collar

**Return to Activity:** If symptoms resolve within minutes and athlete is totally asymptomatic with normal neurologic exam, full strength, and full painless range of cervical motion, may return to sport; recurrent acute and chronic burners are a relative contraindication

## 5.5 CERVICAL INSTABILITY

Clin Sport Med 1998;17:137

**Cause:** Injury and disruption of the ligaments supporting the vertebral bodies

**Epidem:** Potentially catastrophic injury; often due to rapid and excessive/forceful range of cervical motion in one or more planes

**Pathophys:** Injury to the supportive ligaments of the cervical spine with potential for progressive instability, cervical spine deformity, and spinal cord injury; may result in dislocation with compromise of cervical cord; may occur with or without associated cervical fractures and may result in dislocations without associated fractures

**Sx:** Neck pain or stiffness with attempts at extension or flexion

**Si:** Neck pain exacerbated by extension or flexion; may or may not have neurologic deficiencies noted; neurologic findings can vary from weakness to quadriplegia; the presence of bilateral symptoms or lower extremity involvement suggests unstable cervical spine injury

**Crs:** Depends on degree of injury

**Cmplc:** Varying degrees of neurologic dysfunction from mild weakness to complete quadriplegia; can cause catastrophic neurologic injury; muscle spasm may mask abnormal motion

**DiffDx:** Due to severity of injury, if suspected, should rule out instability prior to consideration of other etiologies

**Xray:**
- Radiographs should be obtained
- If radiographs are normal and no fractures, subluxation, or locked facets are identified on routine views, flexion and extension views should be obtained; the athlete should actively flex and extend for these views as tolerated and limited by discomfort or symptoms; pain or neurologic findings limit degree of motion when obtaining these views; athletes that are not alert and oriented should not undergo this examination; rather, they should be immobilized in a cervical collar until mentation is clear

**Rx:** If there exists any suspicion or evidence of cervical instability or neurologic deficits, the cervical spine must be immobilized and the patient immediately transported to appropriate medical facility; the cervical spine should remain immobilized until evaluation by a spine surgeon

**Return to Activity:** Absolute contraindication to contact or collision activities

# 6 Shoulder Injuries

## Acute Injuries

## 6.1 ACROMIOCLAVICULAR SEPARATION

Arch Fam Med 1997;6:376; Med Sci Sport Ex 1998;30(4):S26; Clin
Sport Med 1997;16(4):677; Phy Sportmed 1996;24(3):26; Orthopedic
Sports Medicine, Philadelphia: Saunders, 1994, p 481

**Cause:** Fall or direct trauma

**Epidem:** Common injury in tackling sports (football, soccer, rugby) or
wrestling

**Pathophys:** Tearing of acromioclavicular joint capsule and/or
coracoclavicular ligaments (lateral conoid and medial trapezoid)

*Classification:*

• Grade 1: AC pain without separation/no ligament disruption
• Grade 2: mild separation/AC joint capsule torn, but
coracoclavicular ligaments intact
• Grade 3: Severe separation/AC joint capsule and coracoclavicular
ligaments torn
• Grade 4: grade 3 tear of ligaments with distal clavicle posteriorly
displaced into the trapezius
• Grade 5: grade 3 with severe upward displacement of the distal
clavicle
• Grade 6: grade 3 with the distal clavicle inferiorly displaced and
trapped under the coracoid

**Sx:** Fall on shoulder with arm adducted (at side); pain in the AC area
with or without deformity

**Si:** Tenderness and soft tissue swelling over the AC joint with or
without deformity; positive cross arm test

- Cross arm test: patient standing or sitting, arm forward flexed 90° and internally rotated 90°, examiner forces the arm across the chest (adduction); **Positive test** = pain isolated to the AC joint

**Crs:** Self-limiting pain with residual deformity

**Cmplc:** Brachial plexus injury (stinger/burner), clavicle fracture, rotator cuff tear, acromioclavicular joint osteoarthritis/osteolysis, suprascapular nerve injury

**DiffDx:** Clavicle fracture (see 6.2), coracoid fracture, rotator cuff tear (see 6.4), shoulder dislocation (see 6.3), AC OA (see 6.5)

**Lab:** Consider EMG if suspicion for nerve injury

**Xray:** May be done with or without suspended weights on the arm, rule out coexisting fracture

**Rx:**
- Initial: ice, pain medications, sling for comfort
- Start pendulum ROM activities early as pain will allow
- Shoulder rehab as pain resolves
- Referral to orthopedics for grade 4, 5, and 6 injuries; fracture of distal or medial $^1/_3$ clavicle or humerus; or patient unwilling to accept cosmetic deformity
- Referral to physical therapy for rehabilitation pain modalities in acute and early recovery period

**Return to Activity:** Full ROM without pain; should be able to perform pushups without pain; grade 1, 1–2 weeks; grade 2, 3–4 weeks; grade 3, 4–6 weeks

## 6.2 CLAVICLE FRACTURE

Arch Fam Med 1997;6:376; Clin Ortho 1989;245:89; Phy Sportmed 1999;27(3):119; Orthopedic Sports Medicine, Philadelphia: Saunders, 1994, p 532

**Cause:** Fall onto shoulder with arm at side (adducted) or direct blow

**Epidem:** Football or soccer

**Pathophys:** Most fractures are the middle $^1/_3$

**Sx:** Fall on shoulder or struck by object, audible pop with pain, deformity, and crepitus

**Si:** Loss of motion, gross deformity of clavicle, palpable crepitus, r/o upper extremity neurovascular injury (brachial plexus)

**Crs:** Usually benign in middle $^1/_3$ fractures

**Cmplc:** Brachial plexus injury, delayed or nonunion, open fracture, deformity

**DiffDx:** Grade 3–6 AC sprain with significant clavicular displacement (see 6.1), stinger/burner (see 5.4), coracoid fracture, acromial fracture, sternoclavicular joint subluxation

**Xray:** Classify fracture as medial/lateral/mid $^1/_3$ fracture

**Rx:**

- Figure-of-eight brace for 4–6 weeks
- Pain control (NSAIDs and narcotics)
- Shoulder ROM as tolerated early (pendulum exercises)
- Rehab as pain improves
- Full activity 6 weeks, good strength and full ROM
- Referral for proximal or distal $^1/_3$ fractures, nonunion, evidence of neurovascular injury, patient unwilling to accept cosmetic deformity

**Return to Activity:** At least 6 weeks of rest/immobilization; pain-free ROM and 85% RC strength; normal neuro exam of UE

## 6.3 ANTERIOR SHOULDER DISLOCATION

Arch Fam Med 1997;6:376; Clin Sport Med 1997;16:669; Orthopedic Sports Medicine, Philadelphia: Saunders, 1994, p 580

**Cause:** Fall or direct blow to shoulder

**Epidem:** Anterior dislocation occurs 95% of the time and will be the focus of this discussion; posterior dislocations associated with trauma or seizure

**Pathophys:** The size of the glenoid and humeral head and ROM of the shoulder make it inherently unstable; tear of inferior and middle glenohumeral ligaments and tear or stretch of anterior joint capsule; the "dislocating position" is abduction and external rotation

**Sx:** Fall onto or blow to arm that is abducted and externally rotated; h/o prior dislocation

**Si:** Arm usually held at side adducted and internally rotated; may see or palpate a large infra-acromial sulcus; check distal pulses; check neuro status, especially the sensory distribution of the axillary nerve (posterior deltoid area sensation)

**Crs:** After reduction age <30 with >80% chance of recurrent dislocation; risk of recurrent dislocation in the >40 y/o group is low

**Cmplc:** Instability (recurrent dislocation) (see 6.6); Bankart lesion; adhesive capsulitis (see 6.8); axillary nerve injury; Hill Sachs lesion; missed diagnosis; unable to reduce

**DiffDx:** Humeral fracture, rotator cuff tear (see 6.4), impingement (see 6.7), deltoid strain, biceps tendon subluxation

**Xray:**

- AP and lateral to r/o fracture (may not dx dislocation with these views)
- Axillary or scapular Y view to dx dislocation

  Scapular "Y" is a lateral xray of the shoulder with the arms of the Y formed by the lateral view of the scapular body and the wings or upper arms by the scapular spine posteriorly and the coracoid anteriorly; the glenoid with the overlying humeral head will be in the center

- R/o Bankart lesion: glenoid avulsion fracture from the joint capsule being pulled off seen best in axillary or scapular Y views (it is possible to have a soft tissue Bankart which cannot be see on xray)
- R/o Hill Sachs lesion: posterior humeral head depression from local avascular necrosis due to single or multiple dislocations, seen best with Stryker notch or axillary views

**Rx:**

- Reduction

  Rockwood technique or traction/counter-traction: counter-traction with a towel or strap in the axilla and supported by assistant across the table; gentle traction with internal and external rotation; traction may be made easier by a strap or towel around your waist and the patient's elbow flexed to 90 degrees then lean back to provide gentle traction

  Stimson technique or "hang" method: hang 10–15 lb from arm with patient prone and arm hanging over edge of table; weight should be taped or strapped to the arm; if the patient holds the weight it may increase extremity muscle tone and hinder reduction; hanging over edge of table leave patient undisturbed for 20 min

- Self Reduction of Shoulder Dislocation (Phy Sportmed 2000;28(11):45)

  Pt sits on ground with the ipsilateral knee flexed 90° and both hands clasped around the knee

  The pt leans backward taking slow breaths to allow relaxation of the shoulder muscles and allow reduction

Patients may attempt this technique up to three times before seeking help to reduce the shoulder
- Sedation: IV benzodiazepines (must monitor); 15–20 cc intra-articular lidociane 1%
- Check xrays and neurovascular status after reduction; confirm reduction, look for Bankart lesion; eval axillary nerve function
- Pain control measures, ice and sling immobilization
- Immobilization for short time based on pain (1–2 weeks)
- Even shorter immobilization for older patients
- Begin rehab to strength RC as soon as possible (work on isometrics then isotonics; see 6.4); motion and rehab in frontal plain or across chest is fine; avoid the abducted/externally rotated position (throwing position)
- Referral to orthopedics for inability to reduce, patient <35 (greater chance of repeat dislocation), fracture: humerus, distal clavicle or Bankart lesion, recurrent dislocation

**Return to Activity:** Full, pain-free ROM and normal rotator cuff (RC) strength; negative instability tests (esp. anterior apprehension test; see 6.6)

## 6.4  ROTATOR CUFF TEAR

Arch Fam Med 1997;6:376; JBJS 1989;71-A:499; Am Fam Phys 1996;54:127; Orthopedic Sports Medicine, Philadelphia: Saunders, 1994, p 623

**Cause:** Fall onto shoulder or acute eccentric strain with lift

**Epidem:** More common in the >50 population presenting with shoulder pain

**Pathophys:**
- Functional anatomy: RC = **SITS** muscles (**S**upraspinatus (SS), **I**nfraspinatus, **T**eres Minor, **S**ubscapularis); then tendons of these muscles form a continuous hood over the humeral head; the SS is the major initiator of abduction and the infraspinatus and teres minor or external rotators (ER)
- The RC functions as humeral depressor to keep humeral head in glenoid as power muscles (deltoid, pectoralis major, etc.) move the arm in gross motions

- Weakness and degeneration of the RC (from disuse or sport/occupational overuse) allows upward movement of the humeral head impinging the RC and bursa between the humeral head and acromion
- Degeneration and tearing of the RC occurs in many asymptomatic pts as they age and remain active; symptoms more related to "volume" of the tear (i.e., the size of the hole in the tendon)

**Sx:** History of a fall or lift causing a significant increase in pain and weakness; usually in the dominant arm; h/o shoulder pain with overhead motion of short or long duration; h/o frequent overhead activities

**Si:** Limited motion from weakness or pain; tenderness over anterior rotator cuff(shoulder) area; weak supraspinatus and external rotators; positive impingement signs; may have a positive drop arm test

- Drop arm test: patient standing; fully abduct the shoulder then have the patient slowly lower the arm; **Positive test** = arm suddenly drops to side at about 90° abduction or inability to hold the arm at 90° abduction with minimal downward force applied by the examiner
- Supraspinatus (empty can test) (Fig. 6.1): shoulder abducted 90°, forward flexed 30°, and internally rotated (thumbs down); patient resists downward direct force; compare to opposite side
- External rotation (teres minor and infraspinatus): arm at side and elbow flexed to 90°; patient resists inward directed force; compare sides
- Internal rotation (subscapularis, pectoralis major, latissimus dorsi, teres major): shoulder neutral and elbow flexed to 90°; patient resists outward direct force; hard to isolate the subscap
- Subscapularis lift off: arm maximally internally rotated with back of palm resting in the lower lumbar are; pt attempts to lift the palm of the hand out away from the back against resistance; compare to opposite presumed normal side
- Impingement test (Fig. 6.2): perform Neer and Hawkin's impingement signs (see 6.7) after subacromial injections of lidocaine (see 2.7); if pain relieved but patient still has significant weakness, this is suggestive of a tear

**Crs:** Course depends on the arm dominance, functional activity of the pt (occupation, recreation, hobbies), and the volume of the tear (size of the hole in the tendon)

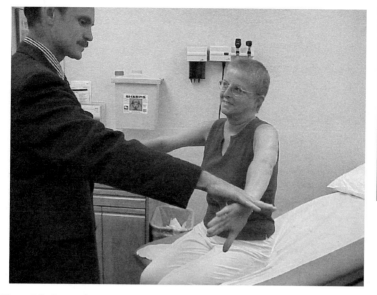

**Figure 6.1.** Supraspinatus strength testing

**Cmplc:** Adhesive capsulitis, glenohumeral (GH) OA, non-repairable tear
**DiffDx:** Rotator cuff tendinopathy (see 6.9), impingement syndrome
(see 6.7), glenohumeral OA, AC OA (see 6.5), C5 or C6
neuropathy/radiculopathy (see 5.3), biceps tendonitis (see 6.10)
**Xray:**
- Plain films usually normal, but may demonstrate arthritis or
spurring of the AC or GH joints
- MRI is not the initial study of choice, must correlate findings with
the clinical exam, may demonstrate rotator cuff tendinosis (increase
signal in the tendon) or tear
- Arthrogram demonstrates leakage of intra-articular contrast into the
subacromial space and will be positive in cases of tear, but cannot
quantitate the size of the tear or diagnose tendinosis
**Rx:** Rotator cuff rehab 1–4 months; pain control medications; activity
modification; consider subacromial injection

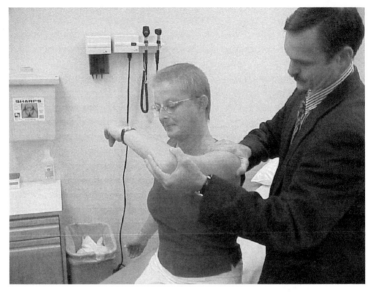

**Figure 6.2.** Hawkin's impingement sign

*Goals:*
- Pain reduction
- Improve range of motion
- Improved strength for ADLs, sport or occupational activities

*Pain Control:*
- Ice (15 min every 2 hrs for 24–48 hrs)
- Modalities: high voltage electric stimulation, iontophoresis, phonophoresis, TENS
- Medications: NSAIDs, Tylenol, narcotics

*Motion:*
- Wall climbs: have patient stand an arm's length from a wall with the affected shoulder closer to the wall; abduct the arm as far as possible; if abduction not full, then complete full abduction by climbing up the wall with the fingers; the patient may need to step closer to the wall as they abduct
- Pendulum exercises: have patient bend forward at the waist with the upper trunk supported by the unaffected arm resting on a low table

or chair; rotate the affected shoulder in slowly enlarging circles to improve range of motion

*Strengthening:*
- Isometric (muscle contraction without motion): early in rehab when pain more severe (abduction, internal/external rotation, forward flexion)
- Isotonic resistance exercise: free weights and weight machines, theraband/tubex (surgical tubing) 12–15 reps × 3 sets 6 sec/rep abduction external/internal rotation, forward flexion

Referral to orthopedics for significant weakness/tear (positive drop arm test), refractory pain and dysfunction/disability, poor response to rehab and observation period (usually >6 months), pt unwilling to accept limitations or disability

**Return to Activity:** Pain-free ROM and 85% strength; may need permanent activity, technique, or equipment modifications

# Subacute and Overuse Injuries

## 6.5 ACROMIOCLAVICULAR OSTEOARTHRITIS

Arch Fam Med 1997;6:376; Orthopedic Sports Medicine, Philadelphia: Saunders, 1994, p 541

**Cause:** Repetitive injury (acute and/or chronic)

**Epidem:** Commonly found on shoulder radiographs although most such AC joint are "noisy" but asymptomatic

**Pathophys:** Chronic overload of joint from overhead/throwing activity and bench press as in wt lifting

**Sx:** Shoulder pain with overhead activities; h/o AC separation or activities with frequent blows to the shoulder or weight lifting

**Si:** Painful crepitus of AC joint with overhead motion; positive cross-chest adduction test with pain isolated to AC joint

**Crs:** Recurrent and unremitting pain with continued activity

**Cmplc:** Subacromial impingement and rotator cuff tendinopathy

**DiffDx:** Osteoid osteoma, undiagnosed clavicle fx (see 6.2), neuralgia from C5 or C6 radiculopathy (see 5.3)

**Xray:** AC joint narrowing with spurring and osteolysis of distal clavicle

**Rx:**
- Symptomatic/pain control
- Activity modification when symptomatic to reduce or avoid overhead activities, weight lifting or pushups
- Trial of 1–2 cortisone injections into the AC joint 6–8 weeks apart
- Referral for refractory pain, unwilling/unable to accept activity restrictions, poor response to injections

**Return to Activity:** Relative pain-free ROM; functionally can do pushups without significant pain

## 6.6 SHOULDER INSTABILITY

Arch Fam Med 1997;6:376; Clin Sport Med 1995;14:761; Clin J Sport Med 1996; 6:40; Orthopedic Sports Medicine, Philadelphia: Saunders, 1994, p 580

**Cause:** Congenital ligament laxity or prior dislocation

**Epidem:** More common in the younger (<30) pt presenting with shoulder pain; most common sports include swimming, tennis, baseball, wrestling, gymnastics

**Pathophys:** Stretched or torn anterior joint capsule and inf and middle glenohumeral ligaments or increased elastin content allowing laxity of multiple joint capsules in the body

**Sx:** Recurrent shoulder pain on the overhead active patient; sense of shoulder "going out"; throwers may complain of "dead arm" symptoms (arm goes dead or numb with a hard throw); h/o prior dislocation

**Si:** May or may not have painful ROM; may or may not have impingement; weakness of supraspinatus and external rotators; positive instability tests (positive anterior apprehension test and relocation test is most common); if 2 or 3 of 3 instability tests are positive check the other shoulder and other joints for laxity

- Instability/tests
  - Anterior apprehension test (AAT) (Fig. 6.3): patient supine at edge of exam table; abduct shoulder to 90° and externally rotate at the elbow while the 2nd hand pushes up (anterior force) on the proximal humerus; **positive test** = pain or apprehension

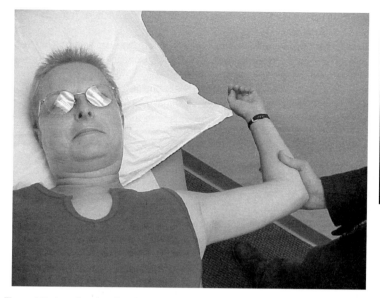

**Figure 6.3.** Anterior apprehension test

indicating a sensation of the shoulder going out or reproducing symptoms

Relocation test: follow the AAT with the relocation test; patient supine at edge of table; abduct shoulder to 90° and externally rotate at the elbow while the 2nd hand pushes down (posterior force); **positive test** = increased tolerance of the external rotation with less or no apprehension; anterior instability is confirmed by a positive AAT and relocation test; positive AAT and negative relocation test may be seen in cases of adhesive capsulitis, rotator cuff tendinosis, or tear and glenohumeral arthritis

Posterior dislocation test (PDT): patient supine with arm forward flexed to 90° and internally rotated 90° with the elbow flexed 90°; apply a posterior (axial) load on the elbow and then cross chest adduct; **positive test** = pain or palpation of a posterior subluxed humeral head or a clunk

Sulcus sign/inferior dislocation test (IDT): patient sitting or standing with the arm hanging at the side; apply axial traction on the arm and observe the infra-acromial space; **positive test** = dimpling indicating inferior displacement of the humeral head and increased acromial–humeral space; this can be quantitated in cm or graded mild, moderate, and severe, and should be compared to the opposite shoulder

**Crs:** Progressive or continued symptoms with high-level sport participation

**Cmplc:** Hill Sachs lesion, GH OA, thoracic outlet syndrome

**DiffDx:** Rotator cuff tendinopathy or tear (see 6.9 and 6.4), labral tear (see 6.11), humeral tumor or cyst

**Xray:** AP, lateral and Y or axillary view to r/o glenohumeral arthritis, Hill Sachs (see 6.3), or Bankart lesions (see 6.3); make sure you order the axillary or Y view

**Rx:** Rotator cuff rehabilitation; activity modification until strong or less symptomatic (avoid threatening positions; i.e., change sport or profile); referral for recurrent symptoms despite rehab or pt unwilling or unable to accept limitations

**Return to Activity:** 85% strength and pain-free ROM; may need modifications of technique or level of intensity to function without pain

## 6.7 IMPINGEMENT AND SUBACROMIAL BURSITIS

Arch Fam Med 1997;6:376; Med Sci Sp Ex 1998;30:S12

**Cause:** Pinching of rotator cuff (RC) and subacromial bursa between acromion and greater tuberosity with abduction

**Epidem:** The most common presentation of primary care shoulder pain

**Pathophys:**
- The RC functions as humeral depressor to keep humeral head in glenoid as power muscles (deltoid, pectoralis major, teres major, latissimus dorsi) move the arm in gross motions
- Weakness and degeneration of the RC (from disuse or sport/occupational overuse) allows upward movement of the humeral head impinging the RC and bursa between the humeral head and acromion

- Additional risk factors related to acromial shape (type I: straight and no risk, type II: semi-curved and mod risk, type III: hooked and high risk) and presence of AC joint spurring from OA with an inferior spur in the subacromial space

Sx: Superior or lateral sharp shoulder pain with overhead activity; may or may not have had prior pain and subacromial injections; usually in the dominant arm; may have night pain

Si: Motion may be limited by pain; AC or subacromial crepitus; positive impingement signs (Neer and Hawkin's); positive impingement test (diagnostic injection) (see 2.7); assess strength of supraspinatus and external rotators; r/o coexistent rotator cuff pathology

*Special tests:*
- Neer impingement sign: patient standing with arm resting at side; examiner internally rotates and forward flexes (elevates) attempting to reach 180°; **positive test** = pain usually noted around 120°
- Hawkin's impingement sign (Fig. 6.2): patient standing or seated with arm forward flexed to 90°, internally rotated 90° with the elbow flexed 90°; the examiner attempts to further internally rotate the shoulder driving the greater tuberosity into the acromion; **positive test** = pain
- Impingement test (diagnostic injection) (see 2.7): perform impingement signs; inject 10 cc of lidocaine 1 or 2% plain per Chapter 2; repeat the impingement signs (Neer and Hawkin's) after 5 min; **positive test** = >50% reduction in pain

Crs: Recurrent episodes common without adequate RC rehab and continued overuse

Cmplc: Chronic pain, RC tear

DiffDx: RC tear (see 6.4), RC tendinopathy (see 6.9), calcific bursitis (see 6.12), cervical radiculopathy (see 5.3), biceps tendonitis (see 6.10)

Xray: R/o AC arthritis with spurring on the underside of the AC joint or acromion; r/o subacromial calcifications

Rx: Activity modification to reduce overhead work; NSAIDs; rotator cuff rehabilitation; trial of subacromial steroid injection (buys temporary relief to allow pt to rehab); referral for significant spurring of the AC or subacromial area, refractory symptoms or suspicion of rotator cuff tear

Return to Activity: Relatively pain-free ROM and 85% strength; may need prolonged recreational or occupational activity restrictions

## 6.8 ADHESIVE CAPSULITIS (FROZEN SHOULDER)

Arch Fam Med 1997;6:376; Med Sci Sport Ex 1998;30:S33

**Cause:** Injury, postop, or idiopathic

**Epidem:** Overall incidence in general population 2–5%; usually 40–70 y/o pt; high incidence in diabetic patients (10–20%) and more common in pts with h/o hyperthyroidism, cervical spondylosis (osteoarthrosis), or reduced motion following injury or bedrest

**Pathophys:** Joint capsule contracture and subacromial and glenohumeral joint adhesions

**Sx:** Painful loss of shoulder motion

**Si:** Limited glenohumeral motion with abduction or forward flexion; very limited Apley's; check active ROM first and follow with passive ROM if not full; range of motion should be compared to the opposite noninjured shoulder; exaggerated scapulothoracic motion for abduction; symptoms generally severe enough that impingement, strength, and instability test cannot be performed

- Normal ROM

| | |
|---|---|
| Forward flexion (elevation) | 0–180° |
| Abduction | 0–180° |
| External rotation | 45° |
| Internal rotation | 55° |
| Extension | 45° |

- **Apley scratch test**: a functional assessment of the ROM; *Apley from below*: the patient attempts to scratch between their scapulae from below; this tests adduction and internal rotation and can be quantitated by the spinal level reached ($T_7$, inf angle of scapula; $T_3$, spine of scapula; $T_2$, superior angle of the scapula) or compared to the opposite shoulder; *Apley from above*: tests abduction and external rotation, which can also be quantitated

**Crs:** Usually will "thaw out" with time

**Cmplc:** Permanent loss of motion, RC tear

**DiffDx:** Glenohumeral OA, RC tear (see 6.4), RC tendinopathy (see 6.9), undiagnosed posterior dislocation, proximal humeral fracture

**Xray:** R/o AC or glenohumeral arthritis or heterotopic calcifications; MRI may need to be performed to r/o rotator cuff tear

**Rx:** The natural history of these shoulders is to improve over time (6–18 months); rotator cuff rehab and formal physical therapy to increase motion; trial of subacromial injection referral for evidence of rotator cuff tear, refractory symptoms after 4–6 months of formal therapy, heterotopic calcifications

**Return to Activity:** Most pts are functional when they can reach the mid lumbar area with the Apley maneuver; pts should have a relative pain-free ROM and 85% supraspinatus strength

## 6.9 ROTATOR CUFF TENDINOPATHY (TENDINOSIS)

Arch Fam Med 1997;6:376; Clin Sport Med 1997;16:674; J Am Acad Orthop Surg 1999;7:32

**Cause:** Overuse

**Epidem:** Common cause of shoulder pain in the middle-aged athlete (30–50); esp. if involved in overhead activities

**Pathophys:** Chronic overuse with tendon degeneration and dysfunction; microscopic exam of tendon demonstrates disorganized fibroblasts (angiofibroblastic hyperplasia; see 7.1)

**Sx:** Shoulder pain with overhead motion of short or long duration; h/o frequent overhead activities; may have a history of a fall causing a significant increase in pain and weakness; usually in the dominant arm

**Si:** Limited motion from weakness or pain; tenderness over anterior rotator cuff (shoulder) area; weak supraspinatus and external rotators; positive impingement signs; in cases of tears, impingement test may relieve pain but patient still has significant weakness

**Crs:** Progressive dysfunction, with recurrent pain episodes/exacerbations

**Cmplc:** Adhesive capsulitis, RC tear, calcific tendonitis

**DiffDx:** Adhesive capsulitis (see 6.8), RC tear (see 6.4), impingement (see 6.7), AC OA (see 6.5)

**Xray:** Usually normal, but may demonstrate arthritis or spurring of AC joint, calcific tendonitis, or bursitis or glenohumeral OA; MRI is not the initial study of choice; must correlate findings with the clinical exam; may demonstrate rotator cuff tendinosis (increased signal in the tendon) or tear

**Rx:**
- Rotator cuff rehab 1–4 months (see 6.4)
- Pain control medications

- Activity modification
- Consider subacromial injection to buy some pain relief to allow pt to continue with rehab
- Referral for refractory pain, poor response to good organized rehab >4 months, evidence of tear, unwilling to accept limitations or disability

**Return to Activity:** Pain-free ROM without impingement and 85% RC strength (supraspinatus and external rotators)

## 6.10 BICEPS TENDONITIS

Arch Fam Med 1997;6:376; Phy Sportmed 1999;27(6):95

**Cause:** Biceps tendon inflammation or subluxation out of the intertubercular groove

**Epidem:** Often associated with RC tear/dysfunction

**Pathophys:** The long head of the biceps assists the rotator cuff as a shoulder depressor and dynamic stabilizer; it passes between the greater and lesser tuberosities in the intertubercular groove and becomes an intra-articular tendon inserting into the superior glenoid

**Sx:** H/o overuse throwing or other overhead activities; similar to rotator cuff tendonosis; pain with overhead motion or shoulder elevation against resistance

**Si:** Anterior shoulder pain; with external rotation the long head in the intertubercular groove can be palpated to be tender
- Speed's test (Fig. 6.4): test for subluxation or tendinitis of the biceps tendon; patient standing and both arms forward flexed 60° in neutral rotation (thumbs up); examiner applies a downward force while the patient resists; **positive test** = pain or giving way (weakness without pain may be noted in old biceps ruptures)
- Yergason's test: tests subluxation or tendinitis of the biceps tendon; patient standing with arm at side and elbow flexed to 90° and forearm neutral (thumb up); patient resists as the examiner extends the elbow and pronates the forearm; **positive test** = pain or pop in the biceps tendon

**Crs:** Chronic pain

**Cmplc:** Rupture

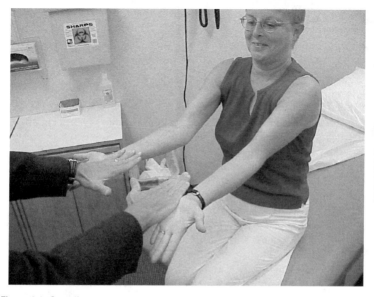

**Figure 6.4.** Speed's test

**DiffDx:** RC tear/tendinopathy (see 6.4 and 6.9), calcific bursitis (see 6.12)

**Xray:** Usually normal

**Rx:** Relative rest from overhead and heavy lifting activities; consider physical therapy modalities for local pain relief; biceps and rotator cuff strengthening; consider local corticosteroid injection with $^1/_2$ cc Celestone and 1 cc lidocaine; referral for refractory pain with rotator cuff dysfunction, evidence of acute or chronic rupture

**Return to Activity:** Pain-free ROM and 85% strength; negative Speed's test

## 6.11 LABRAL TEAR

Arch Fam Med 1997;6:376; Am J Sport Med 1996;24:721; Clin Sport
  Med 2000;19:115; Phy Sportmed 1999;27(6):73
**Cause:** Dislocation, fall, weight-lifting injury
**Epidem:** Common in the younger pt with instability
**Pathophys:**
  • The labrum is a redundancy of the joint capsule as it attaches to the
    glenoid that increases the contact area for the humeral head to
    improve stability
  • Tears usually traumatic: #1 violent eccentric load on the biceps
    tendon avulsing it superiorly creating the SLAP lesion (**S**uperior
    **L**abral **A**nterior **P**osterior); #2 the humeral head levers on anterior
    or posterior labrum with ROM
  • If there is a heavy axial load with this motion, the labrum may be
    torn; #3 traumatic tear with anterior or posterior dislocation
**Sx:** Painful click or pop in shoulder
**Si:** Good ROM and usually good strength; no impingement; may have
    signs of instability (AAT, relocation, PDT, sulcus); positive crank
    or modified crank; positive "SLAPrehension" test
  • Crank test: pt supine with shoulder hanging over edge of table;
    shoulder abducted to 160°; elbow flexed 90° and examiner provides
    axial load on humerus as the humerus is rotated (crank); **positive
    test** = pain with rotation; ± click
  • Modified crank: similar positioning as the crank; examiner now
    provides an axial load/force while the humerus is circumducted
    pinching the labrum 360°; **positive test** = pain and or click when
    the affected part of the labrum is pinched; it is usually good to
    reproduce the symptoms several times for consistency to confirm
  • "SLAPrehension" test (Clin J Sport Med 1998;8(2):121) (Fig. 6.5):
    pt standing and shoulder forward flexed 90° with the elbow
    extended; the examiner performs a cross-chest adduction with
    the forearm suppinated then pronated; **positive test** = pain with
    adduction when arm pronated >> suppinated
**Crs:** Some will become pain free with time
**Cmplc:** Instability; accelerated GH OA
**DiffDx:** Loose body, RC tendinopathy or tear (see 6.4 and 6.9)
**Xray:** Plain films usually normal or may have Bankart or Hill Sachs (see
    6.3); MRI with contrast will demonstrate labral pathology the best

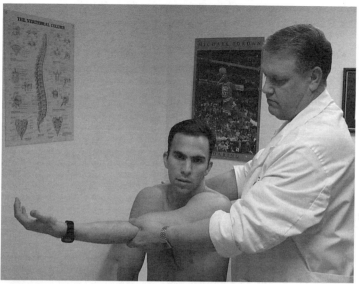

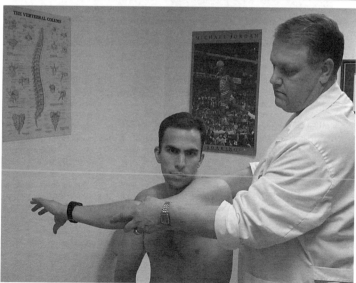

**Figure 6.5A and B**. "SLAPrehension" test

**Rx:**
- RC rehab and observation with activity modification
- Will have problems similar to the pt with instability
- Referral for chronic symptoms, chronic instability, SLAP lesions

**Return to Activity:** Pain-free ROM and 85% strength; asymptomatic instability tests and crank and SLAPrehension tests; functional testing of pushups, throw, and jumping jacks

## 6.12 CALCIFIC BURSITIS AND TENDONITIS

Arch Fam Med 1997;6:376; Phy Sportmed 1999;27(9):27; NEJM 1999;340:1533

**Cause:** Calcium deposition in subacromial bursa

**Epidem:** 30–60 y/o pt; 20–30% bilateral; up to 20% may be asymptomatic

**Pathophys:** Bursal inflammation causing heterotopic calcification that functions as a persistent local irritant or abnormal healing of RC degeneration

**Sx:** Subacromial pain

**Si:** Impingement signs, rotator cuff dysfunction

**Crs:** Usually chronic pain until resolved

**Cmplc:** Chronic pain, RC tear

**DiffDx:** RC tendinopathy (see 6.9), subacromial impingement (see 6.7), fracture (greater or lesser tuberosity), tumor

**Rx:**
- Usually will need aggressive physical therapy
- Rotator cuff rehab for ROM and strengthening
- Subacromial/intralesional steroid injection
- Physical therapy modalities (phonophoresis and US) for mobilization
- Referral to orthopedics for surgical removal if refractory to conservative mgt or evidence of tear

**Return to Activity:** Pain-free ROM and 85% strength and desire to return

# 7 Elbow Problems

## 7.1 LATERAL EPICONDYLITIS/TENDINOSIS (LATERAL TENNIS ELBOW)

JBJS 1999;81-A:259; Clin Sport Med 1992;11:851

**Cause:** Repetitive or overuse injury of the common extensor mechanism: primarily the extensor carpi radialis brevis (ECRB) and sometimes the extensor digitorum communis (EDC)

**Epidem:**
- Higher incidence in athletes >35 yrs, especially those participating in racquet sports; higher activity level (sports or occupational)
- Poor technique; inadequate fitness level

**Pathophys:**
- Repetitive eccentric overload of ECRB and/or the EDC, typically from tennis backhand, leading to degenerative histologic changes within the tendon
- Early reports consistently described this process as inflammatory in nature; however, recent studies have confirmed the presence of fibroblasts, vascular hyperplasia, and disorganized collagen (angiofibroblastic hyperplasia) with a paucity of acute or chronic inflammatory cells, supporting the use of the term "tenidinopathy" instead of "tendonitis"; for further discussion of tendinopathy, refer to Chapter 1

**Sx:**
- Lateral elbow pain typically with activities
- Occasional swelling and weakness of wrist extensors
- Numbness and parasthesias are uncommon

**Si:**
- Focal tenderness to palpation of common extensors overlying the lateral epicondyle

- Typically pain is elicited with resisted wrist extension while the elbow is in full extension, pain with the elbow flexed may indicate more advanced disease
- Pain may also be elicited with resisted supination
- Care should be taken to fully examine the shoulder as well because it is not uncommon to uncover associated rotator cuff weakness

**Crs:**
- Initially pain after activities, which is self-remitting
- Without treatment, pain typically progresses to pain during activities only and may begin to affect ADL and eventually become constant as well as disturb sleep

**Cmplc:** Persistent overload may lead to irreversible tendon damage and possible rupture

**DiffDx:** Cervical radiculopathy at C6–7 (see 5.3); posterior interossseous nerve (PIN) entrapment (see 7.3); radial head fracture; fibromyalgia (if multiple other soft tissue tender points identified); tumor

**Xray:** Calcification or exostosis at the epicondyle or in the tendon close to the tendon attachment may be seen in up to 20% of cases; however, this appears to have no prognostic implications

**Rx:**

*Preventive:*
- Flexibility: stretching exercises for spine, shoulder (including scapula stabilizers: pectoralis, latissimus, rhomboids, trapezius), arm (biceps, triceps), forearm (wrist flexors and extensors)
- Strength: progressive resistive exercise for the shoulder, elbow, wrist, and grip
- Proper technique: strike the ball in front of the body with the wrist and elbow extended, allowing the upper arm and torso, not the wrist extensors, to provide stroke power
- Equipment: lightweight racquet of low vibration material (graphite, epoxies); appropriate grip size (handle circumference should be equal to the measured distance from the tip of the ring finger to the proximal palmar crease, along its radial border); low string tension

*Therapeutic:*
- Protect, rest, ice, compression, elevation, medications, modalities (PRICEMM) (see 1.1)
- Rehabilitation exercises to include: stretching of wrist flexors and extensors; strengthening of wrist, elbow, and shoulder muscles, especially rotator cuff

- Modalities to the affected area (ice, heat, ultrasound, electrical stimulation) with the goal of allowing individual to participate in rehabilitation program; general body conditioning
- Control of force loads as patient returns to activities: counterforce brace (forearm strap); improved sports technique; consider developing a two-handed backhand stroke; control intensity, duration and frequency of activities; appropriate equipment/racquet (see above)
- Consider steroid injection if pain continues to limit participation in rehabilitation program (see 2.6)
- Consider surgery for failure to respond to an appropriate rehabilitation program of 6 months or greater or an unacceptable quality of life

## 7.2 MEDIAL EPICONDYLITIS/TENDINOSIS (GOLFER'S OR PITCHER'S ELBOW)

Am J Sports Med 1994;22:674

**Cause:** Repetitive or overuse injury of the common flexor mechanism: primarily effecting the flexor carpi radialis, pronator teres, flexor carpi ulnaris muscles

**Epidem:**
- Higher incidence in athletes >35 yrs
- Golfers, tennis players, and throwing sports

**Pathophys:**
- Repetitive eccentric overload of common flexors and pronator teres typically occurring in trail arm during a golf swing, forehand in racquet sports, or throwing arm
- Degenerative histologic changes within the tendon: angiofibroblastic hyperplasia (see 7.1)

**Sx:**
- Medial elbow pain typically with activities
- Occasional swelling and weakness of wrist flexors and pronator
- Numbness and parasthesias are uncommon

**Si:**
- Focal tenderness to palpation of over the tip of the medial epicondyle extending distally 1–2 cm
- Often increased pain with resisted wrist flexion and pronation

- May also be associated rotator cuff weakness
- Check for positive Tinel's sign at the cubital tunnel to rule out associated ulnar nerve entrapment (see discussion below)

**Crs:**
- Initially pain after activities, which is self-remitting; progresses to pain during activities only
- Without treatment, pain may begin to affect ADL and eventually become constant as well as disturb sleep

**Cmplc:** Persistent overload may lead to irreversible tendon damage and possible rupture

**DiffDx:** Ulnar (medial) collateral ligament (UCL) sprain or rupture (see 7.6); cervical radiculopathy at C5–6 (see 5.3); ulnar nerve entrapment at the elbow (cubital tunnel syndrome); tumor

**Xray:**
- Calcification or exostosis at the epicondyle or at the tendon attachment
- Calcification within the UCL, may suggest concomitant instability

**Rx:**
*Preventive:*
- Flexibility: stretching exercises for spine, shoulder (including scapula stabilizers: pectoralis, latissimus, rhomboids, trapezius), arm (biceps, triceps), forearm (wrist flexors and extensors)
- Strength: progressive resistive exercise for the shoulder, elbow, wrist, and grip
- Proper technique: for racquet sports see discussion of lateral epicondylitis (see 7.1)
- Equipment: for racquet sports see discussion of lateral epicondylitis; in golf, clubs of proper weight, length, and grip may be selected utilizing the assistance of a golf professional or expert

*Therapeutic:*
- Protect, rest, ice, compression, elevation, medications, modalities (PRICEMM) (see 1.1)
- Rehabilitation exercises to include: stretching of wrist flexors and extensors; strengthening of wrist, elbow, and shoulder muscles especially rotator cuff; modalities to the affected area (ice, heat, ultrasound, e-stim) with the goal of allowing individual to participate in rehabilitation program
- General body conditioning
- Control of force loads as patient returns to activities (counterforce brace; improved sports technique; control intensity, duration, and

frequency of activities; appropriate equipment); see discussion above for racquet sports; improve the golf swing to ensure the swing plane is not too steep (perpendicular to the ground) or too flat (parallel to the ground); consider a graphite shaft and larger heads of golf clubs to minimize vibration forces

- Consider steroid injection if pain continues to limit participation in rehabilitation program
- Consider surgery for failure to respond to an appropriate rehabilitation program of 6 months or greater or an unacceptable quality of life

## 7.3 POSTERIOR INTEROSSEOUS NERVE (PIN) ENTRAPMENT (SUPINATOR SYNDROME, RADIAL TUNNEL SYNDROME)

Electrodiagnostic Medicine, Lippincott-Ravel Pub, 1994, p 891

**Cause:**
- Compression of nerve by lipoma, hemangioma, ganglia, fibroma; missile fragment; laceration
- Fracture and dislocation (*Monteggia fracture*: proximal ulnar fracture with posterior radial head dislocation)

**Epidem:**
- Repetitive wrist use
- 30% of individuals have a sharp fibrous opening of the supinator muscle where the PIN enters

**Pathophys:**
- *Radial tunnel syndrome*: entrapment of the radial nerve where it pierces between the brachialis and brachioradialis before entering the supinator
- *Supinator syndrome*: entrapment of the PIN at the *arcade of Frohse* (fibrous opening in the superficial head of the supinator muscle)

**Sx:** Dull or sharp pain in the extensor muscle mass of the forearm; no sensory loss; weakness of wrist and/or finger extension

**Si:**
- Pain with deep palpation along the proximal radius
- Normal sensory exam, because nerve carries motor fibers

- Radial deviation with wrist extension because of the preservation of the extensor carpi radialis unopposed by the denervated extensor carpi ulnaris
- Weakness and often pain with resisted middle finger extension
- Supination should be checked with the elbow at 90° flexion to help remove the biceps; this may reveal pain and/or weakness

**Crs:** Severe injury may lead to complete wrist drop

**Cmplc:** Without recognition and proper management, irreversible nerve damage may occur

**DiffDx:** Lateral epicondylitis (see 7.1); extensor tenosynovitis; C6–C7 radiculopathy (see 5.3)

**Lab:** EMG/NCV helpful for identifying location and severity of injury

**Xray:**
- Plain films to rule out fracture or exostosis
- CT or MRI to rule out possible mass or space occupying lesion
- Further imaging may also assist with preoperative planning when indicated

**Rx:**
- In the absence of a mass, 8–12 weeks of relative rest should be allowed for spontaneous recovery
- If mass is identified or failure to resolve spontaneously surgery is indicated

## 7.4 OLECRANON BURSITIS

J Accid Emerg Med 1996;13:351; Physical Medicine and Rehabilitation, Saunders Harcourt Health Pub, 1997, p 774

**Cause:** Direct blow or prolonged pressure over the olecranon

**Epidem:**
- One of the most frequently inflamed bursae
- Common in contact sports and in laborers
- More common in males aged 30–60 years

**Pathophys:**
- Inflammatory condition resulting from trauma, infection, or other arthropathy
- Infection typically involves a break of the skin providing a portal of entry of bacteria (*Staphylococcus aureus* representing 90% of cases)

- Permanent damage to the epithelial lining of the bursa predisposes individual to repeated attacks
- Chronic conditions result in thickening and fibrosis of the bursal lining

**Sx:**

- Acute or chronic pain and swelling overlying the olecranon
- Often presents as an acute traumatic episode superimposed upon a more chronic condition

**Si:**

- Palpation of bursal sac reveals tenderness and swelling
- Infection should be suspected with the presence of erythema and warmth
- Range of motion is typically not limited unless extreme elbow flexion causes increased skin tension over swollen bursa
- Fibrous trabeculation within the bursa is often palpated in chronic cases

**Crs:** Recurrence is common

**Cmplc:** Untreated infectious bursitis may lead to sepsis and serious complications

**DiffDx:** Infection: usually *S. aureus*, less common β-hemolytic streptococci; arthritis: manifestation of rheumatoid arthritis or crystalline arthropathy such as gout); fracture; cellulitis; tendinitis (esp triceps)

**Lab:**

- Aspirated fluid should be sent for crystals, cell count, Gram stain, and culture
- Elevated WBC suspicious of infection
- Uric acid if considering gout
- Rheumatoid factor if considering RA

**Xray:** Helpful to rule out possible fracture, calcification, tumor

**Rx:**

- Aspiration should be performed if significant swelling or suspected infections; fluid should be sent to lab and appropriate antibiotic started as indicated
- For noninfectious bursitis, compression and ice packs should be applied
- Heat may apply, particularly after the first 72 hrs to hasten fluid absorption

- Steroid injections should be considered rarely in chronic bursitis as they may cause fat pad atrophy, reducing the natural padding of the olecranon and therefore predispose to recurrent episodes
- Surgical removal of the bursa may be indicated in severe refractory bursitis; appropriate padding of the elbow should be incorporated into primary and secondary prevention

## 7.5 TRAUMATIC ELBOW INJURIES (SPRAIN, STRAIN, FRACTURE)

Phy Sportsmed 1996;24(5):43

**Cause:**
- Collision
- Fall on outstretched arm
- Throwing injury

**Epidem:**
- Contact sports
- Activities at risk of falling (gymnastics, skateboarding)

**Pathophys:** Bony or soft tissue overload.

**Sx:** Acute elbow pain, swelling, reduced range of motion

**Si:**
- Careful palpation for focal areas of tenderness
- Assess for restriction of range of motion (compare to uninjured side)
- Assess for ligamentous stability (ulnar collateral ligament (UCL) stability is checked by applying a valgus stress with the elbow flexed to 20°, radial collateral ligament is checked by applying a varus stress)
- Check for dislocation (usually posterolateral)
- Careful neurovascular examination is imperative

**Crs:** Early recognition and treatment of underlying pathology usually resolves without complications

**Cmplc:**
- Inappropriate diagnosis and treatment may lead to serious deformity and long-term disability
- Failure to recognize neurovascular compromise may result in loss of limb

**DiffDx:** Fracture; dislocation; ligamentous sprain
**Xray:**
- Acute injuries warrant prompt imaging; one should obtain anteroposterior, lateral, olecranon, and occasional oblique views
- *Montaggia fracture*: fracture of the proximal third of the ulna and dislocation of the radial head

**Rx:**
- Although gentle elbow flexion and forearm rotation to a neutral position may result in spontaneous reduction of dislocation, it is best to splint the arm and not move it until the patient can be transported to an emergency room where x-rays may be obtained and the reduction can be performed in a controlled environment
- Immediate reduction may be considered if no medical facility is nearby and neurovascular injury has occurred from fracture or dislocation
- Traumatic injuries leading to ligamentous disruption, fracture, or dislocation warrant immediate splinting and orthopedic consultation

## 7.6 MEDIAL COLLATERAL LIGAMENT (MCL) INSTABILITY

AAOS Instr/course Lect 1999;48:383

**Cause:** Forceful extension of the elbow, accompanied by a valgus stress often created during throwing activities

**Epidem:**
- Sudden traumatic event such as in wrestling or javelin throwing
- Repetitive stress in throwing or overhead sports such as during the volleyball serve

**Pathophys:**
- Acute overload of ligament tensile strength
- Repetitive stress leads to progressive microscopic damage to the MCL

**Sx:**
- Pain along the medial elbow during late cocking or acceleration phases of throwing
- Athlete may experience "opening" or "giving way" of elbow

**Si:**
- Tenderness to palpation along the MCL, particularly at the distal insertion
- Laxity when a valgus stress is applied to the elbow in 20° to 30° of flexion
- *Milking sign*: performed by pulling on the thumb and palpating along the medial collateral ligament while the elbow is flexed, forearm supinated, and shoulder extended; the generation of pain and a sense of laxity indicate a positive sign

**Crs:** Untreated athletes will typically alter their biomechanics promoting further damage

**Cmplc:** Advanced degenerative changes

**DiffDx:** Medial epicondylitis (see 7.2); ulnar nerve entrapment; osteoarthritis

**Xray:** Radiographs will often reveal loose bodies, marginal osteophytes, ligamentous calcifications, or heterotopic bone formation; MRI may help to clarify partial or complete tear of the MCL

**Rx:**
*Preventive:*
- Good throwing mechanics
- Ensure adequate warm-up
- Appropriate conditioning (strength training and aerobic conditioning) to resist fatigue
- Flexibility not only of upper extremities but of trunk, low back and hamstrings as well

*Nonsurgical:*
- Apply principles of PRICEMM (see 1.1)
  Rest may need to extend 2–4 weeks
- Progress to active range of motion when athlete is pain free
- Strength training is added shortly thereafter
- Begin return to throwing program when athlete achieves symmetric range of motion and strength

*Surgical:*
- Indications
  Acute complete rupture
  Chronic pain and/or symptomatic instability that fails to respond to a minimum of 3 months of adequate rehabilitation

# 7.7 DISTAL BICEPS TENDON INJURY

J Am Acad Orthop Surg 1999;7:199

**Cause:**
- Usually a single traumatic event results in overload of tendon, causing avulsion of the tendon from its insertion to the radial tuberosity as well as frequently a tear of the bicepital aponeurosis; all reported cases have involved an extension force with the elbow in 90° flexion

**Epidem:**
- Dominant extremity of males aged 30–60 yrs
- Mean age 50 yrs
- Weightlifting, especially in the presence of anabolic steroid use

**Pathophys:**
- Degenerative changes of the tendon over time compromise the structural integrity of the tendon predisposing it to rupture
- Hypovascularity of the tendon at its insertion has been implicated
- Spurring of the radial tuberosity is common
- An intact bicepital aponeurosis will prevent proximal migration of the ruptured tendon into the arm

**Sx:**
- Sudden sharp, tearing pain in the antecubital fossa or lower anterior aspect of the brachium
- Weakness of elbow flexion and supination

**Si:**
- Ecchymosis in the antecubital fossa
- A visible and palpable defect of the distal biceps muscle is usually obvious in a complete tear
- Incomplete or partial rupture typically reveals crepitus or grinding with forearm rotation
- Weakness with resisted elbow flexion with the forearm supinated
- Weakness with resisted supination with the elbow at 90° flexion

**Crs:** Early recognition and treatment of underlying pathology usually resolves without complications

**Cmplc:** Inappropriate diagnosis and treatment may lead to serious deformity and long-term disability; failure to recognize neurovascular compromise may result in loss of limb

**DiffDx:** Fracture, dislocation, ligamentous sprain

ELBOW PROBLEMS

**Xray:** An MRI is helpful for making or confirming the diagnosis, although not always necessary

**Rx:**

- Complete tears should be treated with early surgical repair, followed by passive range of motion in 4–5 days, then active flexion and extension and forearm rotation in 7–10 days. Light weights (1–2 lb) are introduced in 4–6 weeks; a patient may expect to return to full activities in 3–6 months, depending on the demands of the sport and progress in rehabilitation phase
- Partial and/or incomplete tears may not always require surgery, however, may result in a 20% loss of flexion strength and a 40% loss of supination strength

# 8 Hand Injuries

## Tendon Injuries

### 8.1 MALLET FINGER

Clin Sports Med 1998;17:449
**Cause:**
   • Axial load against an actively extending finger
**Epidem:**
   • Originally described in baseball, but can occur in any activity where the finger is subject to "jamming"
   • Frequently missed initially, with subsequent deformity and medicolegal consequences
**Pathophys:**
   • Can result in a dorsal bony avulsion or a grade III (complete disruption) injury to the extensor digitorum tendon
**Sx:**
   • Pain at the dorsal distal interphalangeal (DIP) joint
**Si:**
   • Inability to extend the isolated DIP
   • Tenderness over the dorsal proximal aspect of the distal phalanx
**Xray:**
   • Bony avulsion from the dorsal proximal distal phalanx seen in approximately 20–30% of cases
**Rx:**
   • Initially treated with PRICEMM (see 1.1) and analgesia as needed
   • No avulsion fracture: splint DIP fully extended for 6–8 weeks straight and an additional 6–8 weeks if engaged in athletic activities
   • Bony avulsion with <30% of joint space involved: dorsal finger splint in full extension for 4 weeks

- Bony avulsion with >30% of joint space involved: refer for possible ORIF
- Permanent DIP extensor lag if untreated; watch for pressure necrosis from splint

**Return to Activity:**

- May return as soon as can be adequately splinted as discussed above

## 8.2 JERSEY FINGER (FOOTBALL FINGER)

Clin Sports Med 1998;17:449

**Cause:**

- Forced extension of the distal phalanx while actively flexing the DIP (e.g., athlete grabbing onto a jersey)

**Epidem:**

- Common in football, rugby, martial arts, or any sport where grabbing an opponent's clothing can occur

**Pathophys:**

- Results in either a grade III tear or a bony avulsion fracture of the flexor digitorum profundus tendon
- An avulsion fracture of the volar lip of the distal phalanx limits retraction and enables repair by ORIF
- Pure tendon avulsions may retract to the proximal interphalangeal (PIP) joint or palm
- If retracted to the palm, the blood supply via the vincula brevum and longum is compromised

**Sx:**

- Pain and swelling at the DIP

**Si:**

- Unable to flex the isolated DIP with localized tenderness at the level of retraction of the avulsed segment
- The flexor digitorum profundus is examined by holding the PIP straight and asking the athlete to flex the DIP
- The superficialis is tested by holding the metacarpal phalangeal (MCP) joint straight and asking the athlete to flex the PIP

**Xray:**

- PA, lateral, and oblique views will document an avulsed fragment and may help localize the level of retraction

**Rx:**
- Initial treatment is PRICEMM (see 1.1) and analgesics as needed
- Refer for surgical repair within 3 weeks with retraction to PIP, within 1 week if retracted to the palm

**Return to Activity:**
- 6–12 weeks following surgery depending on chosen sport

## 8.3 TRAUMATIC DISLOCATION OF THE EXTENSOR HOOD (BOXER'S KNUCKLE)

Clin Sports Med 1998;17:449

**Cause:**
- Caused by direct blow to the flexed MCP or by flexion and ulnar deviation force across the MCP

**Epidem:**
- Collision or contact sports

**Pathophys:**
- Disruption of the sagittal fibers (usually radial) allowing the extensor tendon to sublux off the apex of the MCP into the valley between the MC heads

**Sx:**
- Pain and swelling over the dorsum of the MCP

**Si:**
- MCP is tender dorsally with inability to actively extend the MCP joint from a flexed position
- After passive extension of the joint, the patient is able to maintain extension

**Xray:**
- Plain radiographs usually normal

**Rx:**
- Initially treated with PRICEMM (see 1.1), splinting, and analgesics as needed
- Splint the MCP in full extension with the PIP free for 4 weeks
- Active ROM exercises are begun at 4 weeks with the splint worn at all other times
- Splint is discontinued at 8 weeks
- Old injuries should be referred for possible surgical correction

## 8.4 CENTRAL SLIP AVULSION

Clin Sports Med 1998;17:449

**Cause:**
- Volar directed force on the middle phalanx against a semiflexed finger attempting to extend

**Epidem:**
- Contact and collision sports

**Pathophys:**
- Disruption of the central slip of the extensor digitorum communis tendon over the PIP joint allowing for migration of the lateral bands volar to the axis of the joint (boutonniere deformity)

**Sx:**
- Pain and swelling over the PIP joint

**Si:**
- The PIP is in 15–30 degrees of flexion with point tenderness over the dorsal lip of the middle phalanx
- There is an inability to actively extend the PIP

**Xray:**
- May show an avulsion fracture at the dorsal base of the middle phalanx

**Rx:**
- Initially treated with PRICEMM (see 1.1) as needed
- PIP is splinted in full extension for 4–5 weeks and further protected during sporting activity for an additional 6–8 weeks
- While splinted, the DIP should be allowed to flex to help relocate the lateral bands back to their normal position
- If an avulsion fragment involves >$\frac{1}{3}$ of the joint, the patient should be referred for possible ORIF

**Return to Activity:**
- 4–8 weeks depending on chosen activity

## 8.5 TRIGGER FINGER

Clin Sports Med 1998;17:449
**Cause:**
- Nonspecific flexor tenosynovitis from overdemand

**Epidem:**
- Rowing, rock climbing, or any activity requiring repetitive finger flexion

**Pathophys:**
- Most common in the flexor tendons of the thumb, middle, and long fingers

**Sx:**
- Difficulty straightening involved finger (triggering), especially in AM, variable degree of pain

**Si:**
- Variable amount of tenderness over flexor tendon sheath aggravated by active finger flexion or passive extension; palpable nodule in flexor tendon sheath

**Xray:**
- Radiographs not indicated

**Rx:**
- Early or no triggering: splint finger at night
- Triggering: inject flexor tendon sheath through a mid-lateral approach over distal $1/3$ of the proximal phalanx while the patient resists active flexion; repeat in 6–8 weeks (see 2.2)
- Splint at night

**Return to Activity:**
- As symptoms allow

HAND INJURIES

# Ligament Injuries

## 8.6 COLLATERAL LIGAMENT TEARS

Clin Sports Med 1986;5:757

**Cause:**
- Result from valgus or varus stress to the PIP, DIP, or MCP

**Epidem:**
- Collision and contact sports

**Pathophys:**
- Causes partial or complete tears of the ulnar or radial collateral ligaments

**Sx:**
- Pain and swelling at the involved joint

**Si:**
- Laxity with valgus or varus stress; the joint may be stable or unstable with active flexion and extension

**Xray:**
- May show avulsion fracture from capsular insertion

**Rx:**
- Initially treated with PRICEMM (see 1.1), splinting, and analgesics as needed
- Stable with active ROM: buddy tape finger to finger adjacent to side of injury for 3 weeks
- Unstable with active ROM or obvious angulation: refer for possible surgical repair

**Return to Activity:**
- As symptoms allow, with protective splinting

## 8.7 PIP VOLAR PLATE RUPTURE (WITHOUT DISLOCATION)

Clin Sports Med 1986;5:757

**Cause:**
- Hyperextension injury causing the distal portion of the volar plate to rupture from its attachment to the middle phalanx

**Epidem:**
- Common in volleyball, football, or any sport where the finger is subject to hyperextension

**Pathophys:**
- The loss of the volar stabilizing force of the PIP allows the extensor tendon to gradually pull the PIP into a hyperextension deformity (reverse boutonniere)

**Sx:**
- Pain and swelling at the PIP joint

**Si:**
- The PIP is in varying degrees of hyperextension with maximal tenderness over the volar aspect of the PIP
- With active extension and flexion, the hyperextended PIP often "locks" in the extended position with an inability to initiate flexion

**Xray:**
- PA, lateral, and oblique may show an avulsion fragment at the base of the middle phalanx

**Rx:**
- Initially treated with PRICEMM (see 1.1) as needed
- Extension block splint for 3 weeks with the PIP blocked at 20–30 degrees of flexion, then buddy tape

**Return to Activity:**
- 3 to 6 weeks with protective splint

## 8.8 SKIER'S OR GAMEKEEPER'S THUMB

Clin Sports Med 1998;17:553

**Cause:**

- Hyperabduction of the thumb MCP joint (e.g., the classic fall on a ski pole causing the thumb to be held while the remainder of the hand plunges into the snow)

**Epidem:**

- Initially observed in Scottish gamekeepers who would kill hares by placing the thumb and index fingers around the neck to hyperextend it
- The injury is now almost exclusively traumatically induced in sports such as skiing

**Pathophys:**

- Ulnar collateral ligament sprain—4 classes:
    Type 1: avulsion fx, nondisplaced
    Type 2: avulsion fx, displaced
    Type 3: torn ligament, stable in flexion
    Type 4: torn ligament, unstable in flexion

**Sx:**

- Pain over the UCL area, weak and painful pinch

**Si:**

- Initiated with stress testing
- Tenderness and swelling over the ulnar aspect of the thumb MCP.
- Stress testing should be performed if there is no evidence of avulsion fracture and is performed as follows:
    The area is anesthetized with either a local block or median and radial nerve blocks at the wrist
    The thumb metacarpal is stabilized with one hand and a valgus stress placed on the MCP with the MCP in full flexion; testing is done in full flexion because with extension or slight flexion the normally taut volar plate gives the MCP stability
    Complete rupture (type 4) is suspected if there is angulation 15 degrees > than the normal thumb or an absolute angulation of >35 degrees
    Angulation less than described above is type 3 and considered stable

**Xray:**
- Radiographs performed prior to any stress testing in order to reveal any avulsion fragment; if avulsion fracture evident, stress testing should not be done; displaced fracture >2 mm or rotated fracture should be considered type 4
- Arthrogram will show extravasation of dye in complete ruptures

**Rx:**
- Initially treated with PRICEMM (see 1.1) and analgesics as needed
- Type 1: thumb spica cast with MCP in full extension for 4 weeks
- Type 2: refer for ORIF
- Type 3: thumb spica cast with IP free and MCP flexed 20 degrees for 3 weeks
- Type 4: refer for ORIF

# Fractures

## 8.9 MIDDLE PHALANGEAL FRACTURE

Clin Sports Med 1998;17:491

**Cause:**
- Direct trauma to finger

**Epidem:**
- Collision or contact sports

**Pathophys:**
- Direct trauma or twisting
- The fractures tend to be transverse, generally angulated palmarly, and are often unstable due to the opposing forces of the dorsal extensor tendon and the FDA palmarly

**Sx:**
- Pain and swelling

**Si:**
- Tenderness and swelling over middle phalanx with varying degrees of deformity
- Always check for rotational deformity

**Xray:**
- Radiographs show degree of angulation or displacement

**Rx:**
- Initially treated with PRICEMM (see 1.1) and analgesics as needed
- Stable, nondisplaced, and nonangulated: buddy tape; use thermoplastic splint for sport activity
- Stable, minimal angulation: immobilize with the MCP flexed 70 degrees, PIP flexed 45 degrees, DIP free and buddy taping to control rotation; splint is removed in 3–4 weeks and ROM exercises begun; the splint is worn during sporting activities for an additional 9–10 weeks
- Unstable (displaced, angulated, unable to hold reduction): refer to orthopedics

## 8.10 PIP FRACTURE DISLOCATION

Clin Sports Med 1998;17:491

**Cause:**
- Caused by an axial load on a semiflexed finger

**Epidem:**
- Collision or contact sports

**Pathophys:**
- The middle phalanx shears dorsally, impacting the palmar articular surface of the middle phalanx with the condyles of the proximal phalanx

**Sx:**
- Pain and swelling over the PIP

**Si:**
- Subtle dorsal prominence over the PIP, with localized tenderness

**Xray:**
- Radiographs demonstrate the proximal aspect of the middle phalanx to be dorsally displaced and the palmar articular fragment to be maintained palmarly

**Rx:**
- Initially treated with PRICEMM (see 1.1) and analgesics as needed
- Small fragment without dislocation: buddy tape
- Larger fragment but <40% of articular surface: closed reduction followed by extension block splint with PIP in 30–60 degrees of flexion for 3 weeks
- Fragment >40% of articular surface: surgical consultation for ORIF

## 8.11 PROXIMAL PHALANGEAL FRACTURES

Clin Sports Med 1998;17:491
**Cause:**
- Direct trauma

**Epidem:**
- Collision or contact sports

**Pathophys:**
- Most fractures are spiral or oblique, tend to shorten, and are therefore unstable
- These are difficult to treat due to the compact anatomy of extensor hood, lateral bands, and flexor tendons surrounding it
- Scarring or displacement disturbs the tendon balance

**Sx:**
- Pain, swelling, variable degree of deformity

**Si:**
- Tenderness, swelling, varying degrees of shortening, angulation, or rotation

**Xray:**
- Radiographs will reveal type and extent of the injury

**Rx:**
- Initially treated with PRICEMM (see 1.1) and analgesics as needed
- Fracture stability and early ROM are critical to successful treatment
- Stable fractures: immobilize with wrist in slight extension, MCP in 70 degrees flexion, PIP and DIP joints free, buddy taping to adjacent finger for 3–4 weeks; Buddy taping is then continued until asymptomatic
- Unstable (usual type): refer to orthopedics

## 8.12 METACARPAL FRACTURES

Clin Sports Med 1998;17:491
**Cause:**
- Direct trauma from either an axial load or compressive forces

**Epidem:**
- 5th MC neck fractures common in boxers and martial arts. Can occur in any contact or collision sport

**Pathophys:**
- Neck fractures tend to angulate volarly to a significant degree; shaft fractures are frequently stabilized by the intrinsic muscles
- 60% are angulated >40 degrees and angulation up to 70 degrees does not result in significant functional disability
- The 2nd and 3rd digits are necessary for power grip and much less angulation (<10 degrees) is acceptable here than the 4th and 5th

**Sx:**
- Pain and swelling

**Si:**
- Varying degrees of angular or rotational deformity

**Xray:**
- Radiographs confirm fracture and degree of angulation/displacement

**Rx:**
- Initially treated with PRICEMM (see 1.1) and analgesics as needed
- Reduction technique:
  Fracture site is anesthetized with hematoma block
  The MCP is flexed 90 degrees and the direction and force of the displacement/angulation is reversed
  After reduction, the wrist is placed in a well-molded ulnar gutter splint incorporating the 4th and 5th fingers with the MCP flexed 70 degrees
  Post-reduction radiographs should confirm adequate reduction
  Splint is worn for 4 weeks and early ROM exercises begun to prevent stiffness
- 5th MC neck fractures should be reduced to <40 degrees, esp., in boxers or baseball players who may have significant functional compromise with an angulation of 40 degrees
- 2nd and 3rd MC neck fractures: should be reduced if angulated >10 degrees and casted with the MCP at 70 degrees for 4 weeks
- MC shaft fractures: immobilized with the adjacent finger with the MCP flexed 70 degrees and PIP slightly flexed; splint is removed after 10 days and active ROM exercises begun; the splint is reapplied if the fracture site remains tender
- Unstable fractures should be referred to orthopedic surgeon

## 8.13 CMC FRACTURE DISLOCATION (BENNETT'S FRACTURE)

Clin Sports Med 1998;17:491

**Cause:**
- Axial and abduction forces to the thumb

**Epidem:**
- Collision or contact sports

**Pathophys:**
- The anterior oblique CMC ligament holds the palmar fragment in its normal anatomic position; the abductor pollicis longus pulls the MC shaft fragment radial and dorsal

**Sx:**
- Pain and swelling over base of thumb CMC

**Si:**
- Variable degree of deformity over the thumb CMC

**Xray:**
- PA, lateral, and oblique radiographs will show the palmar fragment ranging in size from a small avulsion fracture to a large triangular fragment

**Rx:**
- Initially treated with PRICEMM (see 1.1) and analgesics as needed
- These are unstable—refer to orthopedics

# Dislocations

## 8.14 DIP JOINT DISLOCATION

Clin Sports Med 1986;5:757

**Cause:**
- Hyperextension, varus or valgus forces

**Epidemiology:**
- Collision or contact sports

**Pathophys:**
- Rare injury due to the short lever arm of the distal phalanx and strong collateral ligaments
- Often are compound dislocations due to the dense cutaneous ligaments that anchor the overlying skin

**Sx:**
- Pain and swelling over the DIP joint

**Si:**
- Dorsal or lateral angulation of the DIP joint

**Xray:**
- Radiographs will show the angulation and associated fractures

**Rx:**
- Initially treated with PRICEMM (see 1.1), splinting, and analgesics as needed
- Reduction technique: anesthetize with digital block; middle phalanx is stabilized with one hand and the dorsal base of the distal phalanx is "pushed" into reduction
- Post reduction, should be splinted in slight flexion for 10–12 days
- The rare irreducible dislocation should be referred for open reduction

## 8.15 PIP DORSAL DISLOCATION

Clin Sports Med 1986;5:757

**Cause:**
- Hyperextension injury with resultant disruption of the volar plate at its attachment to the middle phalanx

**Epidem:**
- Collision or contact sports

**Pathophys:**
- Loss of the volar stabilizing force causes the phalanx to ride dorsally on the proximal phalanx producing a "bayonet" deformity

**Sx:**
- Pain and swelling over PIP

**Si:**
- Deformity and inability to move PIP

**Xray:**
- Radiographs will reveal a dorsally displaced middle phalanx, parallel to proximal phalanx, with some retraction

**Rx:**
- Initially treated with PRICEMM (see 1.1), splinting, and analgesics as needed
- Reduction technique: anesthetize with metacarpal block; middle phalanx is grasped with one hand, giving slight hyperextension of the PIP; the other hand grasps the proximal phalanx and that thumb pushes the middle phalanx into reduction; longitudinal traction of the middle phalanx may allow soft tissue interposition into the PIP and should be avoided
- Post reduction, should be placed in dorsal extension block splint with PIP blocked at 20–30 degrees of flexion but allowed to flex for 3 weeks; follow with buddy taping until symptoms resolve

## 8.16 PIP PALMAR DISLOCATION

Clin Sports Med 1986;5:757

**Cause:**
- Torsional or shearing stress applied to a semiflexed joint

**Epidem:**
- Collision or contact sports

**Pathophys:**
- The above forces result in rupture of one collateral ligament from its proximal attachment and the central slip insertion allowing the proximal phalangeal condyle to buttonhole through the torn extensor mechanism
- The torn collateral ligament may become trapped between the middle and proximal phalanges, preventing closed reduction

**Sx:**
- Pain and swelling over the PIP

**Si:**
- Tenderness over the PIP, especially dorsally and on the side; varying degrees of angular or rotational deformity

**Xray:**
- PA, lateral, and oblique radiographs show volar displacement of the middle phalanx

**Rx:**
- Initially treated with PRICEMM (see 1.1), splinting, and analgesics as needed
- Closed reduction may be attempted, but these are frequently irreducible or unstable; if reduction is successful (post-reduction films show normal congruence of joint surfaces), the treatment is same as for central slip avulsions
- Irreducible dislocations should be referred to orthopedics

## 8.17 MCP DISLOCATION

Clin Sports Med 1997;16:705
**Cause:**
- Torsional or shear forces across the MCP

**Epidem:**
- Collision or contact sports

**Pathophys:**
- Simple dislocations: the volar plate remains attached and the proximal phalanx rests perpendicular to the MC
- Complex dislocation: the MC head goes through the volar plate causing a buttonhole effect, and rests between the lumbricals radially and long flexors ulnarly

**Sx:**
- Pain, swelling, and stiffness at the MCP joint

**Si:**
- Variable degree of deformity
- Simple dislocations: the proximal phalanx is dorsally angulated 60–90 degrees
- Complex dislocations are subtler appearing with the involved digit (usually the index finger) slightly hyperextended and ulnar deviated with dimpling on the palmar surface of the MCP

**Xray:**
- Simple dislocation: lateral view shows hyperextended MCP
- Complex dislocation: PA shows widened joint space with asymmetric inclination of proximal phalanx toward the more ulnar finger; lateral view may show sesamoid interposition between proximal phalanx and MC

**Rx:**

- Initially treated with PRICEMM (see 1.1), splinting, and analgesics as needed
- Simple dislocation—same technique as for PIP dorsal dislocation
- Complex dislocation—reduction may be attempted if injury is acute and no swelling has occurred

    The deformity is exaggerated and the base of the proximal phalanx is pushed over the articular surface; no longitudinal traction is applied as this will tighten the entrapment described under anatomy; once reduced, this is stable and the finger is buddy taped and early ROM begun

    These are generally irreducible and should be referred to orthopedics

# 9 Wrist Injuries

## Fractures and Osseous Injury

### 9.1 SCAPHOID FRACTURE

Clin Sports Med 1998;17:469

**Cause:** Falling on an outstretched hand resulting in hyperextension of wrist

**Epidem:** Most common carpal fracture; accounts for more than 70% of carpal fractures

**Pathophys:**
- Scaphoid bridges proximal and distal carpal rows and serves key stabilizing role in wrist
- Unique blood supply feeds from distal end and results in slower healing in mid and proximal fractures
- Three main types: distal or tuberosity, waist, proximal pole

**Sx:**
- Pain in anatomic snuffbox after appropriate mechanism
- Pain with extension of wrist and firm grip

**Si:**
- Swelling and occasionally bruising is seen
- Marked tenderness to palpation in anatomic snuffbox
- Pain with extremes of extension, flexion, and ulnar deviation

**DiffDx:** De Quervain's tenosynovitis (see 9.5), carpal or carpal-metacarpal DJD, instabilities (see 9.10)

**Crs:** Frequent delayed union or nonunion

**Xray:**
- Initial xray often negative, repeat image in 2 weeks may demonstrate fracture

- Three-phase bone scan will demonstrate occult fracture 72 hours after injury
- MRI can demonstrate fracture earlier

Rx:
- Initial treatment is PRICEMM (protection, rest, ice, compression, elevation, and medications/modalities) and thumb spica splint
- In nondisplaced fracture, thumb spica cast for 6–12 weeks until clinical healing is demonstrated is the rule; sources differ regarding long arm or short arm casting; most typically, long arm for 4 weeks followed by short arm until healed
- Displaced fractures, proximal fractures, and nonunions require surgical pinning

Cmplc: Nonunion requiring surgical fixation

## 9.2 HAMATE FRACTURE

Clin Sports Med 1998;17:469

Cause: Direct blow to hypothenar eminence fractures hook

Epidem: Relatively rare but occurs in baseball, club and racquet sports, and martial arts

Pathophys:
- Most commonly fractured at the hook, which may lead to ulnar nerve injury
- Fracture of the body can occur in conjunction with dorsal metacarpal dislocation

Sx:
- Pain, swelling, and bruising at hypothenar eminence
- May have numbness along fifth digit (deep branch of ulnar nerve)

Si: Tenderness at hamate/hook

Xray:
- Radiographs usually diagnostic; carpal tunnel view for hook fractures, oblique wrist films for body
- CT or tomograms may be useful if not visualized on plain radiographs

Rx:
- Hook fractures often require surgical extraction of hook
- Nondisplaced body fractures treated with short arm cast for 4–6 weeks; displaced fractures require wire fixation

**Return to Activity:**
- Usually can participate with appropriate cast as symptoms allow
- Bracing and physical therapy following casting

**Cmplc:**
- Ulnar nerve entrapment
- Nonunion

## 9.3 LUNATE OSTEONECROSIS (KIENBÖCK'S DISEASE)

Orthop Clin No Am 1986;17:461

**Cause:** Unknown

**Epidem:**
- Associated with repetitive compressive forces (gymnastics, cheerleading)
- Typically in younger athletes

**Pathophys:**
- Micro stress fractures with subsequent loss of blood supply lead to AVN
- Associated with ulnar minus wrist, which increases compressive forces on lunate

    Ulnar minus-distal ulna is shorter that distal radius

    Stahl classifications: stage 1, acute (normal xray, MRI positive); stage 2, sclerotic changes; stage 3, lunate collapse; stage 4, pancarpal arthrosis/instability

**Sx:**
- Initially present with vague aching pain, which increases in severity
- Complain of stiffness
- Usually no history of substantial trauma

**Si:**
- Tenderness at lunate
- Nonspecific painful range of motion

**Crs:** Can continue to progress to complete collapse of lunate with severe arthrosis and carpal instability

**Xray:**
- Initial films are normal or may show nonspecific sclerosis or degenerative cysts; eventually show progressing sclerosis and collapse of the lunate
- MRI is study of choice for early diagnosis

**Rx:**
- Should be immobilized and referred to a hand specialist for evaluation
- Stage 1: lunate decompression through radial shortening or ulnar lengthening procedures; revascularization procedures are also advocated
- Stage 2–3: silicone implant and scaphotrapezial–trapezoid arthrodesis
- Stage 4: proximal row carpectomy

**Cmplc:** Common: Degenerative joint disease with chronic pain and loss of function

## 9.4 DISTAL RADIUS FRACTURE

Clin Sports Med 1998;17:469

**Cause:**
- Falling on an outstretched hand most common
- Also direct trauma or forced wrist extension

**Epidem:**
- Account for >15% of fractures seen in the emergency room
- Common in snow boarders, skating, roller sports, and collision sports

**Pathophys:**
- Extra-articular fractures from relatively low energy trauma generally result in fracture to metaphysis (Colles' fracture)
- Intra-articular fractures are more common in athletes and arise from high-energy axial load; results in four-part comminution in predictable pattern involving radial shaft, radial styloid, dorsal medial fragment, and palmar medial fragment

  The majority of these comminuted intra-articular fractures are unstable and will require specialty consultation

**Sx:**
- Pain, swelling, bruising, deformity at radial wrist
- Numbness, tingling, or dysesthesias may occur

**Si:**
- Tenderness about the distal radius, swelling, bruising, deformity at radial wrist
- Neurologic and vascular exam may demonstrate compromise

**Crs:**
- Stable fractures heal in 4 to 6 weeks with cast immobilization
- Unstable fractures usually require surgical fixation

**Xray:**
- Assess degree of angulation and displacement of metaphyseal fractures
- AP, lateral, oblique generally sufficient to demonstrate intra-articular fractures
- Tomograms are useful to evaluate die-punch lesions of articular radius

**Rx:**
- Stable metaphyseal fractures without angulation can be managed with cast immobilization for 6 weeks; some prefer a long arm for initial 2–3 weeks; serial radiographs should be obtained weekly for the first 3 weeks to ensure no change in alignment
- Angulated metaphyseal fractures tend to be unstable after reduction; these can be treated with a well-molded long arm cast for 4 weeks followed by short-arm for an additional 2 weeks; these fractures must be followed closely for loss of reduction
- Intra-articular fractures are usually unstable and should be seen by an orthopedic surgeon for treatment

**Return to Activity:**
- Usually can return to activity with appropriate cast as symptoms allow
- Bracing and physical therapy following casting

**Cmplc:**
- Fracture at Lister's tubercle associated with rupture of EPL
- Intraarticular fractures associated with degenerative joint disease

# Tendon Injuries

## 9.5 DE QUERVAIN'S TENOSYNOVITIS

Clin Sports Med 1992;11:77

**Cause:** Repetitive wrist motion

**Epidem:** Most common in racquet and throwing sports

**Pathophys:**
- Tenosynovitis of the extensor pollicis brevis or abductor pollicis longus
- Both tendons occupy the 1st dorsal wrist compartment and are generally both involved

**Sx:** Pain and swelling along the radial wrist; pain with gripping and rotational motions (removing the lid from a jar)

**Si:**
- Tenderness along extensor thumb, radial wrist, and forearm
- Pain with resisted thumb abduction or extension
- Finkelstein's test (Fig. 9.1): thumb is passively flexed beneath the flexed fingers and wrist is passively flexed to the ulnar side; a positive test produces pain in the 1st dorsal wrist compartment

**DiffDx:** Scaphoid fracture (see 9.1), carpal or carpal–metacarpal DJD, instabilities (see 9.10)

**Crs:** Can be insidious onset or acute onset associated with specific event; chronic pain is common if untreated

**Xray:**
- Plain radiographs normal
- MRI may be useful to rule out tendon rupture

**Rx:**
- PRICEMM (protection, rest, ice, compression, elevation, medications, physical modalities) for pain relief
- Protective bracing with a thumb spica splint
- Physical therapy to address strength and flexibility issues
- Corticosteroid injection: after sterile preparation, 2 cc betamethasone (6 mg/cc) with 3–5 cc lidocaine is injected into the tendon sheaths within the 1st dorsal wrist compartment (see 2.3)
- Surgical treatment involving a synovectomy may be necessary in persistent cases

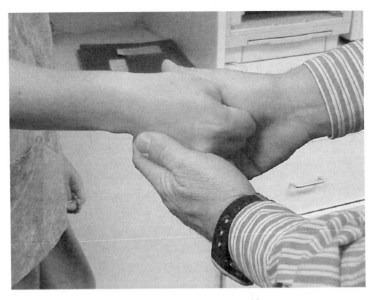

**Figure 9.1.** Finkelstein's test for De Quervain's tenosynovitis

**Return to Activity:** With protective splinting as symptoms allow
**Cmplc:** Chronic pain and dysfunction

## 9.6 INTERSECTION SYNDROME

Clin Sports Med 1992;11:77
**Cause:** Usually from overuse
**Epidem:** Most common in racquet or throwing sports, but can occur
with direct trauma in any activity
**Pathophys:** Intersection comprised of extensor pollicis brevis, abductor
pollicis longus, and the wrist extensors
**Sx:** Pain along dorsoradial wrist; worse with gripping or twisting
motion in wrist

**Si:**
- Tenderness and often swelling along dorsoradial forearm at the junction of the distal and middle thirds
- Pain localized to this area with resisted extension of wrist or abduction/extension of the thumb

**Crs:** Usually insidious onset and chronic symptoms

**Xray:** Plain radiographs normal

**Rx:**
- PRICEMM (see 1.1) for pain relief
- Protective bracing with wrist in neutral or slight dorsiflexion
- Physical therapy to address strength and flexibility issues
- Corticosteroid injection: after sterile preparation, 2 cc betamethasone (6 mg/cc) with 3–5 cc lidocaine is injected into the tendon sheaths at the point of tenderness
- Surgical treatment rarely indicated

**Return to Activity:** With protective splinting as symptoms allow

## 9.7 EXTENSOR CARPI ULNARIS (ECU) TENDINITIS

Clin Sports Med 1992;11:77

**Cause:** Injury from acute strain or repetitive motion injury to ECU tendon

**Epidem:** Most commonly seen in golf, racquet sports, and wrestling

**Pathophys:**
- ECU is contained in the 6th dorsal wrist compartment
- Arises from acute strain or subluxation resulting from eccentric radial deviation or hyper-supination of the wrist, respectively, or repetitive motion
- Often confused with TFCC injury

**Sx:**
- May describe an acute strain injury (such as duffing a ball in golf) or a repetitive activity involving wrist radial/ulnar deviation
- Pain at ulnar wrist exacerbated by wrist extension or ulnar deviation

**Si:**
- Tenderness at ulnar wrist may be hard to distinguish from TFCC tear
- Pain with resisted ulnar deviation and passive radial deviation
- Pain with resisted wrist extension

**DiffDx:** TFCC tear (see 9.11), ulnar styloid fracture, dorsal impaction syndrome (see 9.12)

**Xray:**
- Xrays negative
- MRI may show tenosynovitis and will help distinguish from TFCC tear

**Rx:**
- PRICEMM (see 1.1)
- Bracing
- Corticosteroid injection may be helpful; 2 cc Celestone (6 mg betamethasone/cc) in 3 cc lidocaine is injected into the tendon sheath

**Return to Activity:** With protective splinting as symptoms allow

## 9.8 FLEXOR TENOSYNOVITIS

Clin Sports Med 1998;17:433

**Cause:** Can arise from single eccentric overload event, more commonly from repetitive overuse

**Epidem:** Gripping activities (cycling, racquet sports, batting, and golf)

**Pathophys:**
- Three distinct tendon groups: flexor digitorum, flexor carpi ulnaris, flexor carpi radialis
- Inflammation of the tendons may result in compressive neuropathies (see Chapter 16)
  Flexor digitorum—carpal tunnel syndrome
  Flexor carpi ulnaris—ulnar neuropathy

**Sx:**
- Pain localized to flexor compartment(s), which may include length of forearm; aching pain often at rest following activity
- Pain with active flexion or passive extension of the wrist
- Neurologic symptoms (numbness, tingling) with FD or FCU

**Si:**
- Tenderness localized to involved tendon
- Manual muscle testing produces pain localized to specific tendon
- Neurologic examination may demonstrate compressive neuropathy

**Xray:** Usually normal

**Special Testing:** EMG useful for CTS (flexor digitorum) and ulnar neuropathy (FCU)

**Rx:**
- PRICEMM (see 1.1)
- Bracing or casting (recalcitrant symptoms)
- Physical or occupational therapy to improve ROM and strength; eccentric exercise probably most effective
- Corticosteroid injection:
    CTS (flexor digitorum)—2 cc Celestone (6 mg betamethasone/cc) with 2 cc lidocaine into carpal tunnel (see 2.5)
    Flexor radialis—2 cc Celestone (6 mg betamethasone/cc) with 3 cc lidocaine into the tendon sheath
    Flexor carpi ulnaris—2 cc Celestone (6 mg betamethasone/cc) with 3 cc lidocaine into the tendon sheath
- Surgery: carpal tunnel release; tendon sheath synovectomy for stenosing tenosynovitis

## 9.9 COMMON EXTENSOR TENOSYNOVITIS

Clin Sports Med 1998;17:433

**Cause:** Overuse, infection from penetrating trauma, rheumatologic conditions, and acute strain injury

**Epidem:**
- Less common than other wrist tendinopathies in the athlete
- More commonly related to vocational duties

**Pathophys:** Common extensors reside in the 4th dorsal wrist compartment

**Sx:**
- Painful swelling in dorsal midline wrist
- Pain with motion in the wrist that extends into 4th dorsal compartment of forearm

**Si:**
- "Goose foot sign" erythema and swelling on dorsal wrist and hand involving the tendon sheath of the extensor tendons
- Pain with resisted extension of fingers at the MP joints

**Lab:** Without history of trauma, screening rheumatologic tests indicated including ESR, RF, and ANA

**Xray:** Radiographs negative

**Rx:**
- PRICEMM (see 1.1)
- Neutral wrist splint or casting in recalcitrant cases
- Physical therapy to improve tendon glide and flexibility may be helpful
- Decompressive surgery for stenosing tenosynovitis may be required

**Return to Activity:** As symptoms allow

# Ligament Injuries

## 9.10 SCAPHOLUNATE (SL) DISSOCIATION

Clin Sports Med 1998;17:533

**Cause:** Fall on an outstretched hand

**Epidem:**
- Most common type of carpal instability
- Collision sports, skiing, snowboarding, gymnastics

**Pathophys:**
- Disruption of the scapholunate interosseous ligament
- Allows nonsynchronous movement of the lunate in relation to scaphoid

**Sx:**
- Painful swelling at dorsal wrist
- Painful motion especially with radial deviation of wrist

**Si:**
- Tenderness and swelling at scapholunate articulation
- Watson shift test: examiner places thumb on distal pole of scaphoid on athlete's palm; as the wrist is radially deviated, the normal

scaphoid will flex against the examiner's thumb; in SL instability, the examiner can prevent scaphoid flexion and this is painful

**Crs:** Chronic instability leads to progressive degeneration within the proximal row most noted at radioscaphoid articulation; eventually leading to collapse of scaphoid

**Xray:**
- Initial radiographic findings may be subtle with slight increase in scapholunate space (>3 mm); ring sign: scaphoid is flexed on PA view and will appear short with a ring appearance due to the end-on projection of the cortex
- Lateral view may demonstrate a dorsal intercalated segment instability (DISI) with the lunate dorsally angulated in relation to the scaphoid
- MRI arthrogram of the wrist may be useful to delineate anatomy of the injury

**Rx:**
- Initial treatment with protective splinting, ice, and pain management
- Should be evaluated by a hand surgeon relatively early following injury

**Cmplc:**
- Degenerative joint disease
- Chronic pain

---

# Other Problems

---

## 9.11 TRIANGULAR FIBROCARTILAGE COMPLEX (TFCC) TEAR

Clin Sports Med 1998;17:567

**Cause:**
- Fall on an outstretched hand
- Hyper rotation of wrist or forearm

**Epidem:**
- Degenerative injuries relatively common in gymnasts with ulna plus wrists
- Acute tears with wrist hyperextension (roller sports, collision sports)

- Avulsion injuries with forced wrist rotation (wrestling, golf, racquet sports)

**Pathophys:**
- Degenerative disease from repetitive overload to central TFCC (thinnest portion of complex) due to impaction of triquetrum on ulna
- Acute tear frequently due to compressive forces between the lunate and the ulna in hyperextension injury
- Avulsion of TFCC from ulna (may include ulnar styloid) results from hyper rotational injury

**Sx:**
- Ulnar sided pain following appropriate mechanism of injury
- Swelling and bruising may be seen
- Pain with gripping or manipulation

**Si:**
- Tenderness at carpiulnar interspace
- Pain precipitated with passive pronation, supination, and ulnar deviation; palpable click may accompany pain
- Assess stability of distal radial ulnar joint (DRUJ): Shuck test: examiner grasps radius in one hand and distal ulna in the other; volar directed force is applied to the distal radius and degree of motion is compared to the contralateral side

**Crs:** Frequently results in chronic relapsing ulnar wrist pain

**Xray:**
- Plain radiographs useful to assess ulnar variance and for presence of distal ulnar fracture
- MRI arthrogram can demonstrate tear

**Rx:**
- TFCC tear with DRUJ instability should be managed surgically
- TFCC tear without instability: initially treated with cast or brace immobilization in slight ulnar deviation/flexion for 4 weeks; followed by wrist ROM and strengthening with protective bracing for activities
- Typically seen in the chronic phase without previous diagnosis or treatment; treatment in this case includes 2–4 weeks immobilization; corticosteroid injection is useful for analgesia (6–12 mg betamethasone in 2 cc anesthetic into the carpiulnar interspace) (see 2.4)
- Arthroscopic treatment often required

**Cmplc:** Chronic pain and dysfunction

## 9.12 DORSAL IMPACTION SYNDROME

Clin Sports Med 1998;17:611
**Cause:** Repetitive loading of wrist with super-physiologic loads
**Epidem:** Gymnasts, cheerleaders
**Pathophys:**
- Loaded hyperextension leads to chronic synovitis (meniscoid of the wrist) or microscopic injury to osteocartilage
- Typically involves scaphoid or lunate, which may develop proximal dorsal ridge

**Sx:** Pain with wrist extension
**Si:**
- Tenderness at proximal mid dorsal wrist
- Pain in this area with wrist extension

**Xray:** Usually normal but may demonstrate hypertrophic bone at proximal scaphoid, lunate, or at distal radius
**Rx:**
- Initial treatment involves limitation of hyperextension; a functional brace (e.g., lion's paw) most often successful
- Corticosteroid injection at the site of injury also often helpful, 1 cc (6 mg) betamethasone in 1 cc lidocaine
- Persistent cases may respond to cast immobilization with activity avoidance for 3–6 weeks
- Surgery may be indicated to debride ossicle in chronic cases

**Cmplc:** Degenerative joint disease

## 9.13 WRIST GANGLION

J Am Acad Orthop Surg 1999;7:231
**Cause:** Frequently idiopathic, may arise after trauma (either acute or repetitive)
**Epidem:**
- Most common tumor of the wrist; usually seen on dorsal wrist (scapholunate joint)
- More common in sports with repetitive wrist loading (gymnastics, cheerleading), but seen in athletes of all sports

**Pathophys:**
- Cyst is continuous with joint capsule and is filled with synovial fluid
- Occult ganglia tend to be smaller and more painful; frequently are the cause of vague wrist pain
- Scapholunate joint most common, but can arise from any joint

**Sx:**
- Vague wrist pain may precede appearance of ganglion
- Complain of mildly tender mass that may be reducible

**Si:**
- Mobile mass usually palpable; may be tender
- Typically transilluminate
- Pulsatile mass suggestive of aneurysm and should be further evaluated

**Crs:** May reduce and recur; intermittently tender/painful

**Xray:**
- Usually normal
- MRI may be helpful to evaluate for occult ganglion

**Rx:**
- Aspiration may be attempted but seldom curative
- Surgical treatment for symptomatic ganglia or for cosmesis

# 10 Back Problems

## 10.1 MECHANICAL LOW BACK PAIN (LBP)

Spine 1997;22:2128; JAMA Aug 1992;268:760; U.S. Dept of Health and
Human Services Agency for Health Care Policy and Research,
Number 14, Dec 1994

**Cause:** Repetitive overuse or single event injury (MVA, golf swing, fall,
etc.)

**Epidem:**
- Yearly prevalence of 50%, with 15–20% presenting for care
- 60–90% lifetime incidence
- Most common cause of disability in <45 y/o age group
- 90% recover in 1 month
- Estimated annual cost of $25–100 billion

**Pathophys:**
- Functional anatomy: 5 lumbar vertebrae and discs, posterior facet
  joints, synovial joint that limits extension, longitudinal and
  interspinous ligaments, major muscles include extensors: erector
  spinae, profundi, flexors: abdominal muscles

**Sx:**
- Traumatic injury or fall, MVA, lifting or twisting
- Mild/mod/severe lumbar pain with minimal radiation
- H/o prolonged sitting with work or travel
- No "red flags"
  Fracture: h/o trauma
  Infection or cancer: age >60, weight loss, fever, night pain, h/o
    cancer (bone mets common in breast, lung, thyroid, renal,
    prostate), infection risk factors of IV drug use, immune
    suppression, recent bacterial infection
  Cauda equina syndrome: saddle anesthesia, bowel or bladder
    dysfunction, progressive neurologic deficit

**Si:** Paraspinal muscle tenderness, no bony tenderness, and pain in back with passive knee to chest stretch, negative discogenic exam

**Crs:** 85% of episodes of mechanical LBP will resolve in 12 weeks

**Cmplc:** Prolonged disability for work, recurrent LBP, inability to participate in sport/recreational activity

**DiffDx:** Discogenic back pain (see 10.2), infection, metastatic disease, cauda equina syndrome, fracture (acute-spinous process, compression fx; chronic/subacute-stress fx of pars interarticularis), SI dysfunction (see 10.3); non-back pain (AAA, pyelonephritis, posterior penetrating ulcer, pancreatitis, etc.)

**Lab:** If indicated, consider CBC, ESR, and UA

**Xray:**
- Image if h/o trauma, "red flags," symptoms >1 month
- Lumbar spine series (AP and lateral)
- Bone scan for occult injury or infection
- MRI usually not necessary

**Rx:**

*Acute:*
- Bed rest <48 hrs
- Ice massage (15 min every 2 hrs) followed by passive knee to chest stretch (one leg at a time then both legs together)
- NSAID of choice for 5–7 days
- Short-term use of narcotic pain meds for severe pain
- Valium 5 mg tid for 1–2 days for severe spasm
- Daily walks followed by stretching
- Physical therapy for modalities and stretching: ice massage, electrical stimulation, iontophoresis/phonophoresis

*Subacute:*
- Continued pain management
- Survey for "red flags"
- Stretching of hamstrings and back (knee chest)
- Strengthening of back flexors (abs) and extensors
- Consider low dose TCA (Elavil 10–50 mg hs or Pamelor 10–50 mg hs) for chronic pain and sleep disturbance
- Injection of trigger points (1 cc of 1% lidocaine @ each site)

*Prevention:*
- Aerobic exercise and general conditioning
- Proper lifting techniques

*Referral:*
- "Red flags" to appropriate consultant ASAP
- Physical therapy for rehab and lumbar stabilization program
- Pain clinic for chronic pain management
- Chiropractic for manipulative mgt
- Osteopath for OMT

**Return to Activity:** Activity is the cornerstone of therapy; when pt can tolerate flexion/extension activities, has a normal neurologic exam, and functional performance of gait, lumbopelvic rhythm on FF, and a desire to return to activity, whether it be sport or occupation

# 10.2 DISCOGENIC BACK PAIN

### [Sciatica or Herniated Nucleus Pulposus (HNP)]

Am Fam Phys 1999; 59:575; The Low Back Pain Handbook, Mosby, 1996, p 71

**Cause:** Bending/twisting motion causing herniation of the nucleus pulposis through the annulus fibrosus

**Epidem:**
- Middle aged adults 30–40 y/o
- 95% @ L4–5 and L5–S1
- 75% resolve spontaneously within 6 months
- Cumulative risk of 2nd proven disc during next 20 yrs is 8%
- Most commonly involve L4–5 or L5–S1, with involvement of the L4, L5, or S1 nerve roots

**Pathophys:**
- Functional anatomy: disc with central soft nucleus pulposus and surrounding "onion skin" layers of the annulus fibrosus
- Years of abuse and degenerative change allow cracks and tears in the annulus eventually allowing rupture of the nucleus
- Injury by bending/twisting forces
- Radicular pain probably related to mechanical compression/irritation and chemical irritation of the nerve root

**Sx:**
- Past h/o discogenic or mechanical LBP
- Onset of symptoms with single event bend or twist activity

- Pain usually in the buttock or SI area or leg
- Pain with Valsalva (cough, sneeze, lift, bowel movement)
- Distal neuro complaints of weakness, pain, or paresthesia
- Evidence of bowel or bladder symptoms (urinary retention more common)

**Si:**
- Back usually asymptomatic (if pt has back pain it is probably secondary myofascial pain)
- Pain in sciatic notch ($^1/_2$ way between the greater trochanter and ischium)
- Positive SLR (straight leg raise-pt supine and knee extended, as the leg is elevated between 30 and 70 degrees pain radiating posteriorly below the knee)
- Symptoms aggravated by dorsiflexion of foot
- Distal neuro findings:

|    | Motor | Reflex | Sensory |
|----|-------|--------|---------|
| L3 | Hip flexors | patellar | medial thigh |
| L4 | Tibialis anterior and quads | patellar | medial leg/foot |
| L5 | Extensor hallucis longus (EHL) | none | dorsal foot |
| S1 | Peroneals; foot plantar flexion | Achilles | lateral foot |

Note: test the gastroc-soleus complex by having the patient perform repetitive toe raises and compare to opposite side or may walk in office on heels then toes.
- Spinal reflexes: anal wink, cremasteric, rectal tone

**Crs:** 85% symptomatic discs resolve in 12 weeks with conservative/nonoperative management

**Cmplc:** Permanent nerve damage to spinal root with weakness or paresthesia, chronic pain, central disc/cauda equina

**DiffDx:** Diskitis, compression fracture, spondylosis, mechanical LBP (see 10.1), SI dysfunction (see 10.3), pyriformis syndrome or other gluteal muscular pain, ischial bursitis hamstring pain, gluteal abscess, abdominal path (AAA, posterior perforating ulcer, pancreatitis, etc.)

**Lab:** Usually not necessary

**Xray:** HNP is a clinical diagnosis, radiographs for "red flags" or h/o trauma; MRI should be considered if sx >4–6 weeks, severe motor loss (foot drop or acute quad tone loss); CT imaging can be done but its utility being minimized by the widespread use and availability of MRI

**Rx:**

*Acute:*
- Pain control with NSAIDs and judicious use of narcotics
- Short-term bed rest (<48 hrs)
- Consider short course corticosteroids (hold NSAIDs) (e.g., prednisone 2 mg/kg/d for 5–7 days)
- Stool softener

*Subacute:*
- Increase activity as tolerated
- Monitor neuro exam

*Referral:*
- Symptoms >6 weeks (esp. pain)
- Severe motor loss
- Bowel/bladder dysfunction

**Return to Activity:**
- Pain free with good back motion
- Normal strength or stable strength if there is evidence of motor loss
- Beware of lifting techniques and activities that involve repetitive bending or trunk twisting

# 10.3 SACROILIAC (SI) DYSFUNCTION

Am Fam Phy 1992;46:1459; The Low Back Pain Handbook, 1997, Hanley & Belfus, Inc, Philadelphia, p 91

**Cause:** Acute or chronic injury to sacroiliac joint

**Epidem:** 40% of chronic back pain

**Pathophys:**
- Functional anatomy: SI joint is a biconcave joint connecting the hemipelvis to the sacrum
- The SI joint transmits load from the lower extremities to the spine and it does have movement
- Injury from inflammation, compression/shear forces, hypermobility

**Sx:** May be overuse or repetitive trauma; report of land on single leg stepping off stair or curb with sudden or delayed ipsilateral SI area

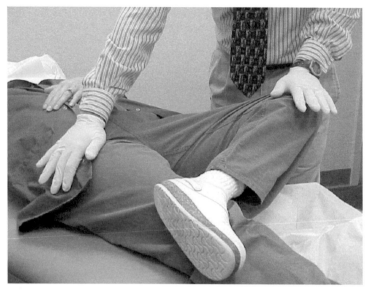

**Figure 10.1.** FABER test for SI pain

pain; pain localized with some radiation into the gluteal area; ± Valsalva symptoms; often cyclic and chronic

**Si:** May have localized soft tissue pain in SI area; absent discogenic signs; positive SI provocative tests:

- FABER: Flexion/Abduction/External Rotation of the hip as in the "figure four" position producing ipsilateral SI pain (Fig. 10.1)
- SI compression: patient on side with affected hip up; downward load applied to the hemipelvis with pain in the affected SI joint
- Gaenslen's: Pt is supine at edge of exam table; the examiner passively flexes one leg to the chest of the pt while the leg near the edge of the table hangs over extending the leg at the hip; pain in the SI of the hip that is extending is positive
- Standing knee to chest: the patient stands on one leg while drawing the other knee to chest; pain in the SI joint of the weight bearing leg is positive

**Cmplc:** Chronic pain and dysfunction

**DiffDx:** Discogenic pain (see 10.2), inflammatory sacroiliitis (spondyloarthropathy), gluteal abscess or muscular strain, pyriformis syndrome, pelvic path (UTI, prostatitis, uterine/ovarian pain radiation, perirectal abscess)

**Lab:** Consider labs to r/o inflammatory process: CBC with diff, ESR/CRP, ANA, RF, UA; ? value of HLA-B27 as screening test

**Xray:** SI views for signs of displacement, sclerosis, or degenerative change; bone scan for evidence of inflammation in chronic symptoms; MRI for follow-up eval

**Rx:**
*Acute:* Similar to mechanical LBP
- Ice
- Knee–chest stretch
- NSAIDs
- Prn short-term narcotics
- Soft tissue injections

*Subacute:*
- SI self-mobilization
- Physical therapy for modalities and manipulation

*Chronic:*
- SI injection under fluoroscopy
- OMT/chiropractic manipulation
- Self-mobilization

*Referral:*
- Physical therapy for modalities
- Pain clinic for injections and pain modalities
- OMT/chiropractic
- Rheumatology for evidence of inflammatory arthritis

**Return to Activity:** Negative or normal provocative tests; tolerance to trial of activity (walking, running, lifting)

# 10.4 LUMBAR SPINAL STENOSIS

Am Fam Phys 1998;57:1825; Clin Orthop 1992;279:82; Rheum Dis Clin North Am 1994;20:471

**Cause:** Progressive spondylosis (degenerative arthritis of disc and facet joints) causing compression of spinal cord and nerve roots

**Epidem:** 1/100 >65 undergo laminectomy annually for this problem

**Pathophys:** Functional anatomy: osteophyte formation and synovial hypertrophy as well disc narrowing that contribute to narrowing of the spinal canal and neuroforamina

**Si:** Arthritis with morning stiffness or stiffness after inactivity; back or lower extremity (unilateral or bilateral) with prolonged standing or extension activities (walking downhill, down stairs or looking overhead); relief with sitting for short periods of time; may or may not have bowel or bladder symptoms; rare Valsalva symptoms; ?? distal neuro sx

**Sx:** Limited back motion by pain and arthritis (esp. in extension); exacerbation of symptoms with extension double leg or single leg; absent SLR; absent SI provocative tests; may have distal neuro findings (see 10.2); look for absence of anal reflex

**Crs:** Progression of symptoms is common; degree of impairment and rate of progression is variable

**Cmplc:** Irreversible neurologic deficit; chronic pain requiring escalating narcotic pain meds

**DiffDx:** Metastatic disease, discogenic pain (see 10.2), infection, compression fx, spondylosis, retroperitoneal path (PUD, pancreatitis, AAA, pelvic path, pyelonephritis)

**Lab:** Usually not necessary except to work up the diff dx

**Xray:** Lumbar osteoarthritis on radiograph with evidence of spurring, spondylolisthesis (anterior or posterior), disc narrowing, or neurforaminal narrowing; MRI more definitive imaging study (with or without intrathecal contrast); CT generally not helpful

**Rx:**

*Acute:*
- Limit standing/extension activities (stair/hill descent)
- Programmed rest stops if have to be on feet
- NSAID or COX-2 inhibitor
- Short-course corticosteroid for severe radicular symptoms

*Subacute/Chronic:*
- Epidural steroid injections (ESI)
- Flexion-biased rehabilitative exercises
- Cushioned shoes/insoles
- Low impact aerobics
- Bike, stairmaster, aqua-aerobics

*Referral:*
- Anesthesia pain for ESI (usually a series of 3 injections)
- Neurosurgery for refractory pain or bowel/bladder/motor symptoms in pt with good operative risk

**Return to Activity:** Long-term management should try to limit high impact activity and depending on symptoms, avoid repetitive bending and twisting

# 11 Hip and Thigh Problems

## Anterior Hip and Groin

### 11.1 FEMORAL STRESS FRACTURE

Int J Sports Med 1993;14:347; Skeletal Radiol 1986;15:133; Clin Orthop 1994;303:155

**Cause:** Typically follows change in training volume or intensity

**Epidem:** Most common in running sports; amenorrheic females are particularly susceptible

**Pathophys:**

- Imbalance between osteoblastic and osteoclastic cell activity with bone reabsorption outpacing bone formation leading to weakening of cortex
- Femoral neck injuries classified as distractive (superior cortex) and compressive (inferior cortex)
- Related to intrinsic factors (foot mechanics, poor flexibility, muscle imbalance, coxa vara, etc.) and extrinsic factors (running surface, shoe selection, etc.)

**Sx:** Vague, increasing groin or thigh pain, made worse with activity; late finding is pain with active hip flexion and at rest

**Si:**

- Tenderness in the affected groin
- Pain with a single leg stance
- Passive internal rotation of the hip is painful
- Pain with active hip flexion common late finding

**Crs:** Insidious onset with gradual worsening pain; if untreated, can result in frank fracture; return to activity time variable

**DiffDx:** Femoral head avascular necrosis (see 11.2), acetabular labral tear (see 11.3), adductor strain/tendonitis (see 11.5), iliopectineal bursitis (see 11.4), iliopsoas tendon strain (see 11.6), osteitis pubis (see 11.7)

**Xray:**
- Plain radiographs are usually normal in early stress reaction, may demonstrate cortical sclerosis or frank fracture in later studies
- Triple phase bone scan is very sensitive even in early stress fractures
- MRI is useful in diagnosing stress fractures and may be less expensive than bone scan

**Rx:** Based on location of injury
- Femoral neck-distraction cortex: treat aggressively and refer early, usually require surgical treatment
- Femoral neck-compression side: the main treatment is rest followed with periodic plain radiographs to document healing
- Crutch ambulation with toe to floor weight bearing for 6–12 weeks is the norm
- Physical therapy directed at improved flexibility and balanced muscle strengthening should be employed as symptoms allow
- These patients should be referred to an orthopedic surgeon if symptoms persist, there is evidence of fracture on plain radiograph, or if there is evidence of avascular necrosis on any study
- Femoral shaft and pubis stress fracture treatment includes rest and activity substitution using pain as a guide (advise the patient to exercise to pain not through pain); rarely require surgical intervention

**Return to Activity:** Minimum of 6 weeks are required before the patient can gradually resume normal weight-bearing activity

## 11.2 FEMORAL HEAD AVASCULAR NECROSIS

Orthopedics 1994;17:789; Semin Arthroplasty 1991;2:241

**Cause:** Most often not identified

**Epidem:** Predisposing factors include: prolonged corticosteroid use, heavy alcohol abuse, stress injury, or fracture; over 50% are idiopathic

**Pathophys:** Loss of normal vascular watershed involving all or part of femoral head resulting in tissue death

**Sx:**

- Insidious onset of atraumatic groin and anterior leg pain
- Present at rest, worse with activity
- May be bilateral

**Si:**

- Tenderness in the affected groin
- Pain with a single leg stance
- Passive internal rotation of the hip is painful

**Crs:** Typically progressive pain and development of DJD

**Cmplc:** Degenerate joint disease with limitation in function and chronic pain

**DiffDx:** Femoral stress fracture (see 11.1), acetabular labral tear (see 11.3), adductor strain/tendonitis (see 11.5), iliopectineal bursitis (see 11.4), iliopsoas tendon strain (see 11.6), osteitis pubis (see 11.7)

**Xray:**

- Plain radiographs normal early, later demonstrate sclerosis, progressive cortical flattening, and degenerative joint disease
- MRI will demonstrate early disease prior to radiographic changes

**Rx:**

- Early surgical intervention is possible including cortical drilling and vascularized bone grafting; results vary
- Symptomatic treatment for pain relief
- Activity modification
- Total hip arthroplasty for late DJD

# 11.3 ACETABULAR LABRAL TEAR

Orthopedics 1995;18:753

**Cause:** Twisting injury on weight bearing hip

**Epidem:** Incidence unknown; most common in collision sports

**Pathophys:**

- Tear of the fibrocartilaginous ring around peripheral acetabulum
- Recently described entity thought to be responsible for many cases of chronic anterior hip pain

**Sx:**

- Deep, anterior hip pain, typically described as sharp or stabbing
- May or may not have history of macro-traumatic event
- Pain is worse with activity

Si:
- May not have tenderness on palpation
- Often, pain with passive external or internal rotation
- Thomas flexion-to-extension test: patient lies on the contralateral side with both hips maximally flexed; the affected hip is then moved from full flexion to full extension; painful click suggests labral tear

Crs: Frequently, chronic anterior hip pain not responsive to treatment; may resolve with decreased activity

DiffDx: Femoral stress fracture (see 11.1), femoral head avascular necrosis (see 11.2), adductor strain/tendonitis (see 11.5), iliopectineal bursitis (see 11.4), iliopsoas tendon strain (see 11.6), osteitis pubis (see 11.7)

Xray:
- Plain radiographs normal
- Diagnostic lidocaine injection (intra-articular) alleviates pain temporarily
- MRI arthrogram may demonstrate tear
- Diagnostic arthroscopy is the gold standard

Rx:
- Trial of PRICEMM (see 1.1)
- Arthroscopy in cases with persistent pain

## 11.4 ILIOPECTINEAL BURSITIS

J Rheumatol 1995;22:1971
Cause: Overuse injury
Epidem: Most common in running, dancing, martial arts
Pathophys:
- Bursa in the deep anterior soft tissues between the iliopectineal eminence and iliopsoas muscle/tendon
- Inflammation related to overuse, poor flexibility, and abnormal gait mechanics

Sx:
- Gradual onset of deep anterior hip pain
- Exacerbated with activity, particularly with hip extension

**Si:**

- Tenderness may be reproducible
- Limp is common
- Pain with active internal rotation and passive extension of hip

**Crs:** Insidious onset, persistent symptoms

**DiffDx:** Femoral stress fracture (see 11.1), femoral head avascular necrosis (see 11.2), acetabular labral tear (see 11.3), adductor strain/tendonitis (see 11.5), iliopectineal bursitis (see 11.4), iliopsoas tendon strain (see 11.6), osteitis pubis (see 11.7)

**Xray:** Plain radiographs usually negative; MRI may demonstrate fluid in bursa or inflammatory changes of the iliopsoas tendon

**Rx:**

- PRICEMM (protection, rest, ice, compression, elevation, medications, and modalities)
- Physical therapy to address flexibility and gait issues
- Surgery has been described

## 11.5 ADDUCTOR TENDON STRAIN

Am Fam Phys 1999;60:1687

**Cause:** Acute strain injury

**Epidem:** Most common in collision or contact sports

**Pathophys:** Injury to adductor muscle group caused by eccentric external rotation with hip in abducted position

**Sx:**

- Abrupt onset of sharp pain in groin following appropriate injury
- Continued pain with ambulation, kicking, and jumping

**Si:**

- Point tender in groin
- Pain elicited with passive abduction, active adduction, and resisted internal rotation

**DiffDx:** Femoral stress fracture (see 11.1), femoral head avascular necrosis (see 11.2), acetabular labral tear (see 11.3), iliopectineal bursitis (see 11.4), iliopsoas tendon strain (see 11.6), osteitis pubis (see 11.7)

**Xray:** Plain radiographs rule out avulsion injury

**Rx:**
- PRICEMM (protection, rest, ice, compression, elevation, medications, and modalities)
- Stretching and strengthening exercise within limits of pain

**Return to Activity:** Gradual return to full activities in 1–4 weeks with augmented stretching program for prevention

## 11.6 ILIOPSOAS TENDON STRAIN

Am Fam Phys 1999;60:1687

**Cause:** Acute strain injury

**Epidem:** Common in soccer and football

**Pathophys:** Eccentric strain injury caused by forceful contraction of iliopsoas with the foot planted or with hip in extended position

**Sx:**
- Abrupt onset of groin pain with appropriate mechanism
- Pain with active hip flexion (walking or running)

**Si:**
- Tenderness in affected groin
- Pain with passive external rotation and active hip flexion

**Crs:** Acute onset, fairly debilitating

**DiffDx:** Femoral stress fracture (see 11.1), femoral head avascular necrosis (see 11.2), acetabular labral tear (see 11.3), adductor strain/tendonitis (see 11.5), iliopectineal bursitis (see 11.4), osteitis pubis (see 11.7)

**Xray:** Plain radiographs may reveal avulsion fracture from the lesser trochanter in young patients

**Rx:**
- Initial PRICEMM (protection, rest, ice, compression, elevation, medications, and modalities)
- Early range of motion within pain-free range
- Structured therapy for improving strength and flexibility as symptoms allow

**Return to Activity:** Return to activity in 1–6 weeks

## 11.7 OSTEITIS PUBIS

Sports Med 1991;12:266

**Cause:** Repetitive overload to pelvis (running, jumping, etc.)

**Epidem:**
- Most common in women after childbearing
- Running, jumping, cutting, and collision sports

**Pathophys:**
- Inflammation at the symphysis pubis articulation
- May be related to early return to sports in postpartum period or repetitive macrotrauma leading to relative dynamic instability

**Sx:** Gradually worsening midline groin pain, worse with activity

**Si:**
- Point tender at symphysis pubis
- Pain in midline with single-leg stance

**Cmplc:** Chronic pain

**DiffDx:** Femoral stress fracture (see 1.1), femoral head avascular necrosis (see 11.2), acetabular labral tear (see 11.3), adductor strain/tendonitis (see 11.5), iliopectineal bursitis (see 11.4), iliopsoas tendon strain (see 11.6)

**Xray:** Plain radiographs may show degenerative changes at synchondrosis; bone scan useful to determine active vs. inactive disease at symphysis

**Rx:**
- Relative rest until asymptomatic avoiding precipitating activities
- Nonsteroidal anti-inflammatories
- Corticosteroid injection: 2 cc betamethasone (6 mg/cc) in 3 cc topical anesthetic instilled sterilely into articular space

**Return to Activity:** When asymptomatic

# Lateral Hip

## 11.8 GREATER TROCHANTER BURSITIS

Mayo Clin Proc 1996;71:565

**Cause:** Direct trauma or overuse in the setting of SI dysfunction

**Epidem:** Common in runners, cross-country skiers, and sedentary individuals

**Pathophys:**
- Irritation of any of three bursa overlying the superior margin of the greater trochanter
- Usually due to tightness in IT band, arising from poor flexibility, SI dysfunction, leg length discrepancy, or gait anomalies
- Results from acute trauma, overuse, or mechanical factors including shortened hip abductors or external rotators, increased varus angulation of the hip due to leg length discrepancy, or a broad pelvic structure
- Calcific bursitis is rarely seen

**Sx:**
- Deep, aching, lateral hip pain that may extend into the buttocks or down into the lateral knee
- Pain is aggravated by activity, local pressure or stretching, often worse at night

**Si:**
- Palpation over the bony prominence of the greater trochanter and slightly inferiorly or posteriorly elicits tenderness
- Pain with resisted hip abduction and external rotation as well
- Leg length discrepancy common
- SI tenderness and restricted motion are common
- Ober's test positive: patient lies on unaffected side, both hips and knees initially flexed, affected hip and knee are extended stressing soft tissues over greater trochanter (Fig. 11.1)

**Crs:** Frequently chronic or recurrent lateral hip pain

**Cmplc:** Chronic pain

**DiffDx:** Snapping hip syndrome (see 11.9), hip pointer (see 11.10), neuropathies involving the lumbar nerve roots (L2–4) and branches of the iliohypogastric or subcostal nerves, sclerotomal

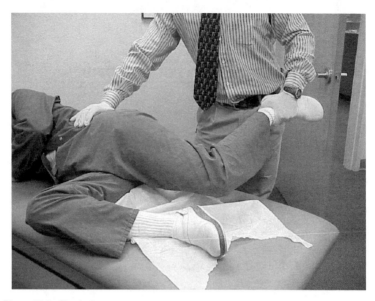

**Figure 11.1.** Ober's test

irritation of lumbar facet joints and paraspinal ligaments, and femoral head and neck pathology (see 10.2, 11.1, 11.2)

**Xray:** Plain radiographs usually normal

**Rx:**

- PRICEMM (protection, rest, ice, compression, elevation, medications, and modalities)
- Rehabilitative exercises aimed at improving flexibility of the iliotibial band, SI function, and hip rotator strength
- Weight loss, conditioning, and proper lifting technique can aid in preventing recurrent or chronic injury
- The local injection of corticosteroid is often effective in relieving symptoms; because of the relatively large volume of this bursa, 10 cc of lidocaine with 80 mg of triamcinolone should be injected at the point of maximal tenderness (see 2.8)

**Return to Activity:** As symptoms allow

## 11.9 SNAPPING HIP SYNDROME

JBJS 1991;73-B:253

**Cause:** Soft tissue friction over the greater or lesser trochanter

**Epidem:** Relatively uncommon; more frequent in female runners, hurdlers, and gymnasts

**Pathophys:** Most commonly related to snapping of iliotibial band over greater trochanter (lateral snapping hip) or the iliopsoas tendon snapping over the lesser trochanter

**Sx:** Painful snapping sensation with hip flexion/extension; groin pain with medial snapping hip syndrome

**Si:**

- Prominent palpable or audible snap with hip flexion and extension
- May reproduce symptoms with flexion, abduction, external rotation (FABER) position (Fig. 10.1)
- Ober's test may be positive (Fig. 11.1)

**Crs:** Often not painful but disturbing to athlete; response to therapy variable

**DiffDx:** Trochanteric bursitis (see 11.8), hip pointer (see 11.10), neuropathies involving the lumbar nerve roots (L2–4) and branches of the iliohypogastric or subcostal nerves, sclerotomal irritation of lumbar facet joints and paraspinal ligaments, and femoral head and neck pathology (see 10.2, 11.1, 11.2)

**Xray:** Normal

**Rx:**

- Physical therapy to improve flexibility and balance rotator strength
- Correct gait abnormalities
- Surgery has been described (z-plasty), not commonly done

**Return to Activity:** As symptoms allow

## 11.10 HIP POINTER

South Med J 1983;76:873, 878

**Cause:** Contusion to ASIS due to direct blow

**Epidem:** Most common in football, hockey, and other collision sports

**Pathophys:** Soft tissue and bone bruising at the site of impact

**Sx:** Pain and bruising following an appropriate mechanism

**Si:**
- Tenderness at ASIS
- Pain with hip abduction or flexion

**Crs:** Symptoms generally resolve in 2–6 weeks

**Cmplc:** Possible development of myositis ossificans (see 11.15)

**DiffDx:** Trochanteric bursitis (see 11.8), snapping hip syndrome (see 11.9), neuropathies involving the lumbar nerve roots (L2–4) and branches of the iliohypogastric or subcostal nerves, sclerotomal irritation of lumbar facet joints and paraspinal ligaments, and femoral head and neck pathology (see 10.2, 11.1, 11.2)

**Xray:** Plain radiographs to evaluate possible fracture of iliac apophysis

**Rx:**
- Rest and protection
- Ice early, heat in sub-acute phase
- Return to activity as symptoms allow (days to weeks)

**Return to Activity:** As symptoms allow, 1–3 weeks

# Posterior Hip and Buttocks

## 11.11 PIRIFORMIS SYNDROME

Orthopedics 1998;21:1133

**Cause:** Symptoms arise from muscle spasm, insertional inflammation, or by irritation of sciatic nerve

**Epidem:** Most common in cyclists and roller sports, more common in females

**Pathophys:**
- Piriformis muscle originates at the sacrum and inserts on the greater trochanter and functions in external rotation of the hip
- The sciatic nerve lies deep to the muscle and may pass through the muscle belly in up to 15% of athletes

**Sx:**
- Aching pain in buttocks often with sciatica
- Worse with prolonged sitting or riding

**Si:**

- Marked tenderness over gluteal prominence
- Pain with resisted abduction and external rotation of the hip and passive internal rotation of the hip (examined with the patient lying and knee in full extension)
- Normal neurologic examination but positive straight leg raise

**Crs:** Chronic, waxing and waning symptoms

**Cmplc:** Chronic pain

**DiffDx:** Ischial bursitis (see 11.12), sciatica/lumbar disk disease (see 10.2), and sacroiliac dysfunction (see 10.3)

**Xray:** Not indicated for piriformis syndrome; lumbar spine x-rays and MRI may rule out lumbar DJD or disk disease as a cause of sciatica

**Rx:**

- PRICEMM (protection, rest, ice, compression, elevation, medications, and modalities)
- Deep tissue massage
- Physical therapy to improve flexibility and correct underlying SI dysfunction
- Chiropractic or osteopathic treatments frequently helpful
- Corticosteroid injection may be helpful but must be approached with caution
- Padded seat for cyclist

## 11.12 ISCHIOGLUTEAL BURSITIS (WEAVER'S BOTTOM)

Am Fam Phys 1996 15;53:2317

**Cause:** Inflammation of this bursa is associated with chronic and continuous direct stress

**Epidem:** Occurs most frequently in sedentary occupations

**Pathophys:** The bursa lies deep to the gluteus maximus over the ischial tuberosity

**Sx:** Complain of pain in ischium with sitting and walking

**Si:**

- Tenderness over the ischial tuberosity
- Exacerbated by passive flexion and resisted extension of the hip

**Crs:**
- Chronic pain
- Symptoms usually relieved with treatment

**DiffDx:** Piriformis syndrome (see 11.11), sciatica/lumbar disk disease (see 10.2), and sacroiliac dysfunction (see 10.3)

**Xray:** Negative

**Rx:**
- PRICEMM (protection, rest, ice, compression, elevation, medications, and modalities)
- Rehabilitation through improving flexibility and strength
- Lifestyle or occupational modification to decrease the direct pressure on this area
- If vocational demands require continued sitting, a foam pad or air filled "doughnut" to decrease direct pressure over the affected ischial tuberosity should be used

# Thigh

## 11.13 MUSCLE STRAINS

J Am Acad Orthop Surg 1998;6:237

**Cause:** Occurs due to a single macro traumatic injury or from repetitive overuse

**Epidem:** Hamstring muscle/tendon injuries are extremely common

**Pathophys:** The most common site of injury is the musculotendinous junction

**Sx:**
- The presenting symptoms depend on the mechanism of injury
- Acute strains present with severe pain following a definable event such as a sprint or jump
- An overuse injury will have a gradual onset of pain which eventually prevents running or other activities

**Si:**
- Tenderness at the musculotendinous junction, which is made worse with active contraction of the muscle

- Swelling, calor, and in the case of muscle tear, ecchymosis and a palpable defect are often seen

Crs:
- Acute injuries resolve in 1–4 weeks
- Overuse injuries can result in chronic recurrent symptoms

Xray: MRI documents location and extent of injury but seldom required

Rx:
- Relative rest, avoiding activities that exacerbate the symptoms until the pain resolves, usually 1–4 weeks
- An aggressive stretching program aimed at the hamstrings, quadriceps, and calf should be instituted as symptoms allow
- The adjunctive use of NSAIDs, ice, ultrasound, and electrical stimulation is useful for pain relief

Return to Activity: 1–4 weeks

## 11.14 MUSCLE CONTUSIONS

Am J Sports Med 1991;19:299

Cause: The usual mechanism is a direct blow

Epidem: The most common examples in the hip and thigh region are quadriceps contusions and injuries to the ASIS (hip pointer)

Pathophys: Direct trauma results in bleeding and swelling into the muscle or periosteum

Sx:
- Complains of pain and bruising following appropriate mechanism
- Pain with active contraction of affected muscle group

Si:
- Localized tenderness, swelling, and ecchymosis at the site
- Pain with passive stretch of affected muscle
- Palpable muscle defect or bruise

Crs: Full recovery is normal in 1–4 weeks

Cmplc: Myositis ossificans (see 11.15)

Xray: MRI can delineate any tear or defect in the muscle

Rx:
- PRICEMM (protection, rest, ice, compression, elevation, medications, and modalities)
- For quadriceps contusion in the acute setting, an elastic wrap should be applied to the leg and calf with knee flexed 120° to hold

the quadriceps in a stretched position for 12–24 hrs; this will limit the loss of flexibility in this muscle
- These injuries should be treated with a gentle stretching program with a return to activity as soon as symptoms allow

**Return to Activity:** Full recovery in 1–4 weeks

## 11.15 MYOSITIS OSSIFICANS (MO)

Orthop Rev 1992;21:1319

**Cause:** Myositis occificans most commonly follows a quadriceps contusion or severe hamstring injury with deep tissue bleeding

**Epidem:**
- Collision sports (football, hockey, rugby)
- Quad compartment and post thigh are most common but has been reported in many areas

**Pathophys:**
- Represents metaplastic formation of bone in the muscle
- Is most likely to arise following repetitive trauma

**Sx:** History of substantial muscle injury followed by persistent painful mass in area of trauma

**Si:**
- Firm mass typically palpable
- A gradual muscle contracture may occur with limited range of motion at the adjacent joints

**Crs:** Bony mass develops 4–6 weeks following injury

**Xray:** Radiographs demonstrate early calcium deposition followed by bone formation in the soft tissues

**Rx:**
- Treatment of myositis ossificans includes a prevention of repetitive injury
- Aggressive stretching and strengthening is advocated by some authors, others suggest absolute rest with early findings of MO
- Surgical release of the mature ossificans sometimes required

## 11.16 AVULSION INJURIES

Skeletal Radiol 1994;23:85

**Cause:** Avulsion fractures about the pelvis occur following an acute, forceful contraction against fixed resistance

**Epidem:** These are most common in the skeletally immature athlete; several tendon insertion sites are commonly involved including:
- Sartorius avulsion from the anterior iliac crest (ASIS)
- Rectus femoris at the anterior inferior iliac spine
- Hamstring origin at the ischium
- Iliopsoas at the lesser trochanter
- Piriformis at the greater trochanter

**Sx:** Sudden pain at the insertion site with swelling, ecchymosis, and tenderness

**Si:** Active muscle testing will significantly exacerbate the patient's pain

**Xray:** Radiographs are usually diagnostic for these injuries

**Rx:**
- PRICEMM (protection, rest, ice, compression, elevation, medications, and modalities)
- Cautioned against challenging the affected muscle to the point of pain for 4–6 weeks
- Structured flexibility and strengthening program should be instituted as soon as symptoms allow
- Surgical treatment may be required with significant displacement of the avulsed segment in iliopsoas or ischial injuries

# 12 Knee Problems

## Acute Injuries

### 12.1 ANTERIOR CRUCIATE LIGAMENT (ACL)

Am J Knee Surg 1998;11(2):128

**Cause:** Mechanism of injury is direct blow to the lateral, medial, or anterior aspects of the knee causing valgus or varus strain, twisting (rotational), or hyper-extension

**Epidem:**
- Varies by activity; alpine skiing; 7/1000 skier days, collegiate football: 5/1000 player days, general population: 3/1000 knee injuries
- Women appear to have increased risk in some sports compared with men; thought to be related to: increased Q angle (formed by line from ASIS to center of patella and line from tibial tuberosity to center of patella), narrower femoral notch, and smaller diameter ligament

**Pathophys:**
- Major stabilizer preventing anterior translation of the tibia with respect to the femur, secondary rotational stabilizer
- Injuries to other intra-articular structures (menisci, collateral ligaments) are commonly associated

**Sx:**
- Patient typically describes a substantial trauma to the knee and often reports hearing or feeling a pop
- Followed (within 2 hs) by a massive joint effusion (hemarthrosis)
- Pain is diffuse
- In chronic injuries, often complain of instability with quick turns or pivot movements

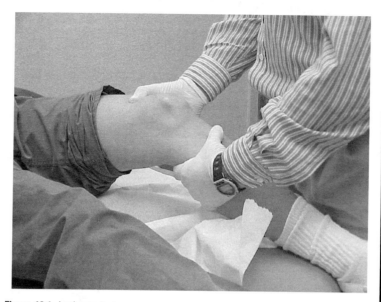

**Figure 12.1.** Lachman test

Si:

- Acutely, substantial intra-articular effusion is palpable, joint line or posterior tenderness is common
- Patency of neurovascular structures should be assessed
- Lachman test: the patient is supine and relaxed, the knee is flexed to 20°, stabilize the distal femur with one hand while exerting an anteriorly directed force on the proximal tibia; excessive anterior translation of the tibia when compared to the uninjured knee indicates instability (Fig. 12.1)
- Pivot shift: the patient is supine and the leg extended with the foot internally rotated, a valgus force is applied at the knee as the knee is slowly flexed; at approximately 30°, a rotatory clunk will indicate a positive test

Cmplc:

- Chronic instability with premature degenerative joint disease
- Instability predisposes to additional acute injury to meniscal cartilage, bone, or ligamentous structures

**DiffDx:**
- Other causes of hemarthrosis: fracture, PCL (see 12.2), MCL (see 12.6), LCL (see 12.7), patellar dislocation (see 12.4), meniscal tear (see 12.3)
- Other causes of instability: PCL, MCL, LCL, patellar dislocation

**Crs:**
- Acute symptoms subside over 4–6 weeks, effusion may persist for 8–12 weeks
- Instability and re-injury of intra-articular structures common
- With recurrent instability, gradual degenerative disease is common

**Xray:**
- Radiographs will occasionally demonstrate a Segond lesion (avulsion fracture at the lateral proximal tibia)
- MRI is confirmatory but not always necessary, however is useful to evaluate for other associated intra-articular injuries

**Rx:**
- Initial: knee immobilizer for 24–72 hs, with crutch ambulation; PRICEMM (protection, rest, ice, compression, elevation, medications, modalities) is useful for symptom relief; structured therapy program should be instituted early to limit strength loss and maintain range of motion
- Subacute: structured therapy including proprioception training and strengthening; functional bracing for activities
- Surgery: indication for surgery is persistent instability; determinants include: age, chosen sport, level of participation, response to therapy; surgery is usually delayed 2–6 weeks after injury

**Return to Activity:**
- Non-operative treatment, graded return to sport over 6–12 weeks
- Surgical treatment, return to play 6–12 months following surgery

---

# 12.2 POSTERIOR CRUCIATE LIGAMENT (PCL)

Am J Knee Surg 1996;9:200

**Cause:** Direct blow to the anterior aspect of the knee (as in a motor vehicle accident), extreme flexion, or anterior directed stress with the knee in full extension (usually results in combined ACL/PCL injury)

**Epidem:**
- Much less common than ACL injuries
- Most common in football and hockey
- NFL draftees have approximately 2% incidence

**Pathophys:**
- Arises anteriorly on the medial femoral condyle in the intracondylar notch; the fibers blend with the posterior capsular fibers at its insertion on the proximal posterior tibia
- The complex biomechanical architecture primarily functions to prevent posterior translation of the tibia with respect to the femur
- The PCL also limits hyperextension and internal rotation

**Sx:**
- Acute: pain in the posterior/lateral knee, swelling, and occasionally, instability with deceleration motions (as in walking down stairs)
- Chronic: instability

**Si:**
- Posteriolateral tenderness, effusion; positive instability testing
- Posterior drawer sign: with the patient supine, flex the hip to 45° and the knee to 90° with the foot flat on the table, a posteriorly directed force is applied to the proximal anterior tibia; increased translation indicates PCL injury
- Sag sign: with the patient supine, the hips and knees are flexed to 90° with both feet supported above the table, a torn PCL will allow the tibial to translate posteriorly in this position in comparison to the uninjured knee.

**Cmplc:**
- Chronic instability leads to early DJD
- Instability can result in injury to other intraarticular structures, including: bone, meniscal cartilage and other ligaments

**DiffDx:**
- Other causes of hemarthrosis [fracture, ACL (see 12.1), MCL (see 12.6), LCL (see 12.7), patellar dislocation (see 12.4), meniscal tear (see 12.3)]
- Other causes of instability (ACL, MCL, LCL, patellar dislocation)

**Crs:** Instability may develop late (years after injury)

**Xray:** Radiographs usually negative; MRI typically diagnostic

**Rx:**
- Initial and non-operative treatment as for ACL injuries
- Reconstruction of PCL injuries is less common than for ACL tears, but may be indicated if instability persists following conservative treatment

## 12.3 MENISCUS INJURIES

J Anat 1998;193:161

**Cause:**
- Twisting injury with the foot planted, valgus or varus strain, hyperextension, or hyperflexion
- Often, the trauma will appear minor or no specific event is recalled on history

**Epidem:**
- Approximately 60 per 100,000 general population
- Most common in cutting sports, football, soccer, basketball, wrestling

**Pathophys:**
- Two "C" shaped fibrocartilagenous structures anchored via the capsule to the tibial plateau
- They are thinner (and thus avascular) centrally, with the periphery relatively well vascularized
- Function in both load sharing to dissipate forces on the proximal tibia, and in maintaining joint integrity

**Sx:** An appropriate mechanism may be described, mild to moderate swelling, joint line pain, pain with flexion or extension, and a sensation of locking or catching within the knee joint

**Si:**
- Effusion, joint line tenderness, and painful passive range of motion; positive meniscal signs
- McMurray's test: with the patient supine, the hip is flexed to 90° and the knee maximally flexed, the examiner then internally or externally rotates the tibia and extends the knee while exerting a valgus or varus force respectively at the knee; McMurray's test is positive if these maneuvers produce a painful pop

- The Apley's compression test: with the patient supine the knee is flexed to 90° and a load is applied to the tibia while the tibia is internally and externally rotated; this will cause pain with a damaged meniscus

**Cmplc:**
- Meniscal degeneration
- Degenerative joint disease

**DiffDx:**
- Other causes of joint swelling (fracture, ligament injury, DJD)
- Other causes of locking or catching (patellar dysfunction; see 12.8)
- Other medial or lateral pain entities (ITB friction syndrome; see 12.14)

**Crs:** Acute symptoms (pain with weight bearing, swelling, painful ROM) last 2–3 weeks with gradual improvement over 8–12 weeks

**Xray:**
- Plain radiographs are negative
- MRI scan is useful for confirming diagnosis, but unnecessary if clinical evaluation conclusive

**Rx:**
- Nonoperative treatment is effective in 50–75% of patients with an uncomplicated meniscal tear
- Initially, PRICEMM measures (see 1.1) with activity modification including short-term crutch use and limited walking for 3–5 days will reduce pain symptoms
- Following the initial rest period, the patient should initiate exercise aimed at maintaining strength and flexibility while limiting pain; alternate activities include cycling, walking, and pool running or swimming
- As symptoms resolve, a gradual running program can be instituted with low intensity, short runs without hills or turns; cutting and twisting activities should be avoided for 8–10 weeks
- If symptoms fail to resolve in 6–12 weeks, the patient should be referred for diagnostic imaging (MRI) or surgical evaluation
- In a mechanically locked knee (i.e., a loss of motion due to meniscal impingement), referral for urgent reduction or surgery should be arranged

**Return to Activity:** As outlined above

## 12.4 PATELLAR DISLOCATION AND SUBLUXATION

Acta Orthop Scand 1997;68:419
**Cause:**
- The most common mechanism is a twisting or valgus motion with a forceful quadriceps contraction
- May be caused by direct blow to medial patella

**Epidem:** Reported in a wide variety of sports; most frequent in jumping and contact activities

**Pathophys:**
- The patella usually dislocates laterally, over the femoral condyle
- This displacement may be a true dislocation, or may be partial, which spontaneously reduces (patellar subluxation)
- Predisposing factors include quadriceps muscle imbalance (VMO hypoplasia with vastus lateralis hypertrophy), patella alta, hypoplastic femoral condyles, increased Q angle, and other functional malalignment

**Sx:**
- Report a sensation of the lateral patellar displacement
- In subluxation, the patella spontaneously reduces as the knee is extended
- Substantial pain, locking, and swelling are common

**Si:**
- If dislocation is seen acutely, the knee is held in flexion with the patella easily palpable on the lateral aspect of the joint
- The orientation of the patella should be determined to plan reduction
- Following subluxation, a large effusion is common and the soft tissues medial to the patella (the retinaculum) will be tender to palpation
- Lateral patellar pain is also common
- Apprehension test: in patients with spontaneous reduction or subluxation, patellar stability is assessed by placing the patient supine with the knee flexed over the examiner's thigh (approximately 10°). The examiner applies pressure to the medial patella forcing it laterally, pain and increased motion are suggestive of patellar instability (Fig. 12.2)

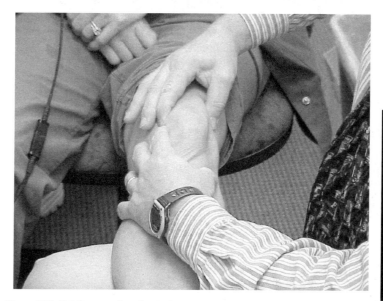

**Figure 12.2.** Patellar apprehension test

**Crs:** Dislocation requires reduction; following reduction, pain at medial retinaculum and lateral patella subsides over 4–8 weeks

**Cmplc:**
- Premature degenerative joint disease

**Xray:**
- Radiographs should be obtained to rule out evidence of fracture or loose body
- MRI is useful to exclude other intra-articular injury

**Rx:**
- If the patient presents with acute patellar dislocation, reduction can be attempted by extending the knee while applying gentle pressure to the lateral edge of the patella
- Following the reduction, the knee should be immobilized for 6 weeks in full extension with a padded knee immobilizer or cylinder cast
- These patients will require aggressive physical therapy to regain full function after prolonged immobilization

- In subluxation without frank dislocation, short-term immobilization until pain resolves (2–4 weeks) followed by physical therapy aimed at VMO strengthening and improved flexibility will generally be effective
- This is followed by the use of a patella brace (open patella knee sleeve) and activity modification as needed
- Surgery may be required in patients with recurrent patellar dislocations

**Return to Activity:** 2–8 weeks depending on severity of symptoms and response to therapy

## 12.5 QUADRICEPS/PATELLAR TENDON RUPTURE

Orthop Clin North Am 1992;23:613

**Cause:** Most commonly injured through an eccentric overload event with a forceful quadriceps contraction in landing (deceleration), jumping (acceleration), or through a direct blow

**Epidem:** Most frequent in sports with extreme eccentric overload (jumping, weight lifting, and football); associated with corticosteroid injections to the patellar tendon

**Pathophys:**
- The extensor mechanism includes the quadriceps muscle group and linkage to the proximal tibia (quadriceps tendon-patella-patellar tendon-tibial tubercle)
- Disruption can occur at any point along this kinetic chain

**Sx:**
- The patient will usually describe an appropriate mechanism
- Painful swelling anteriorly
- Weakness in standing or ambulation

**Si:**
- Frequently, a defect in the extensor mechanism can be palpated
- Swelling, tenderness, and an intra-articular effusion are generally present
- Extensor lag sign: patient will be unable to maintain knee extension against gravity or actively extend from a flexed position

**Crs:** Requires surgical repair

**Xray:** Plain radiographs may demonstrate patellar fracture, tibial tubercle avulsion or tendon avulsion from the patellar poles; MRI is very useful in localizing and grading severity of injury

**Rx:**
- Initial treatment is immobilization in full extension
- Surgical consultation within 24–48 hours

**Return to Activity:** 12–16 weeks following surgical repair and therapy

## 12.6 MEDIAL COLLATERAL LIGAMENT (MCL)

Sports Med 1996;21:147

**Cause:** A valgus stress applied to the lateral knee either through direct blow or noncontact rotational stress

**Epidem:** Common in cutting and contact sports such as soccer, football, and basketball; most common knee ligament injury in female alpine skiers

**Pathophys:** These injuries are graded on a scale of 1 through 3; grade 1 injury denotes a strain without disruption of the ligament (a simple stretch injury), grade 2 injury involves partial disruption of the ligament, and grade 3 injury is a complete disruption

**Sx:**
- Patients will complain of medial joint pain following an appropriate mechanism
- Pain will extend to distal medial femoral condyle or proximal tibia; pain is worse in full extension or flexion beyond 90°
- Initially, swelling may be minimal due to disruption of capsule; swelling is common after the first 24 hours
- In complete disruption, may experience symptoms of valgus instability

**Si:**
- Medial joint line tenderness that extends above or below the joint to the origin or insertion of the ligament
- Moderate effusion common
- Passive range of motion is painful at full extension or flexion beyond 90°.
- Valgus stress test: with patient supine, the knee is flexed to 20°, a valgus strain is applied while maintaining a fulcrum at the lateral

knee; this will produce pain at the medial knee and with a complete tear, medial joint space opening

- Anterior drawer: the patient is supine with the knee flexed to 90° and the tibia placed in external rotation; with a complete tear, the medial tibial plateau will rotate anteriorly when an anteriorly directed force is applied to the posterior proximal tibia

**Crs:**
- Grade 1 injury: return to activity 1–2 weeks
- Grade 2 injury: return to activity in 3–6 weeks
- Grade 3 injury: return to activity in 6–12 weeks

**Xray:** Plain radiographs are non-diagnostic in MCL injuries, valgus stress radiographs will often document instability but are not routinely obtained; MRI will often document location of injury and can distinguish grade 3 injuries from less severe strains

**Rx:**
- Low grade injuries: crutch ambulation, rest, ice, NSAIDs, and functional bracing with a full ROM to relieve acute symptoms
- Rehabilitative exercises should be instituted as symptoms resolve; the patient should be started on alternative exercise activities, such as bicycling, as soon as possible, and resume running as symptoms allow; advise the patient to run on flat surfaces avoiding any quick turns or cutting activities until symptoms completely resolve
- Grade 3 injuries are treated are treated as above except initial immobilization should restrict patient to 30° from full extension (extension block); this is maintained for 2–4 weeks
- Functional rehabilitation including strengthening and flexibility work should be started as symptoms subside
- MCL bracing should be maintained throughout rehabilitative process
- With persistent instability or pain, further evaluation is indicated to rule out other intra-articular injury
- Surgery may be required if instability persists following rehabilitation or if indicated for associated injuries to the ACL, LCL or menisci

**Return to Activity:**
- Low grade injuries may return to activity in 1–2 weeks if effectively braced
- Higher grade injuries, especially in contact sports, require 6–10 weeks to return to activity.

# 12.7 LATERAL COLLATERAL LIGAMENT (LCL)

Sports Med 1990;9:244

**Cause:** These injuries usually occur with a varus strain, twisting, or hyperextension injury

**Epidem:** Less common than MCL injury; common with other significant ligamentous injury of the knee

**Pathophys:** Ligament arises on the lateral femoral condyle and inserts on the fibular head; it is a component of the arcuate complex serving to reinforce the posterior $1/3$ of the capsule and serves as a primary varus restraint. Complete LCL disruption is rarely an isolated injury, frequently associated with complete ACL tear, arcuate ligament complex injuries, and injury to other intra-articular structures

**Sx:**

- These patients will complain of lateral joint pain with symptoms above or below the joint line at the insertion of the ligament
- They may complain of instability with pivoting or twisting activities
- Swelling and bruising are common

**Si:**

- Tenderness at the lateral joint line with extension to the ligament insertion above or below the joint
- Intra-articular effusion is common
- Careful assessment of other intra-articular structures is key
- Varus stress test: the knee is held at 20° flexion and a varus force is applied with the examiner's body while using the hand as a fulcrum on the medial joint space; this will produce pain or an opening in the joint; these injuries are graded 1–3 similarly to MCL injuries
- Anterior drawer: the patient is supine with the knee flexed to 90° and the tibia placed in internal rotation; with a complete tear, the lateral tibial plateau will rotate anteriorly when an anteriorly directed force is applied to the posterior proximal tibia
- Should be assessed for rotatory instability (see ACL/PCL above)

**Crs:** Low grade injury similar to low grade MCL injury; higher grade injuries with instability often require surgery

**Xray:** Radiographs may demonstrate capsular avulsion injury; MRI typically diagnostic

**KNEE PROBLEMS**

**Rx:**
- Low grade strains without evidence of other injury can be managed in the same manner as an MCL injury
- Injuries involving complete disruption of the LCL, posterolateral rotatory instability, or evidence of other intra-articular injury should be referred for orthopedic surgery evaluation

**Return to Activity:**
- Low grade injuries may return to activity in 1–2 weeks if effectively braced
- Higher grade injuries, especially in contact sports or those requiring surgery, require significantly longer to return to activity

# Chronic Knee Problems

## 12.8 RETROPATELLAR KNEE PAIN (PATELLOFEMORAL PAIN)

Orthopedics 1997;20:148

**Cause:** Overuse syndrome in setting of knee malalignment

**Epidem:** This is the most common cause of chronic anterior knee pain in the young athlete

**Pathophys:**
- Etiologic factors are described as intrinsic, those related to anatomy, and extrinsic or external factors
- Intrinsic factors include patellar malalignment [increased Q angle (see 12.1), patella alta or baja, lateral patellar tilt], quadriceps muscle imbalance, poor hamstring and quadriceps tendon flexibility, iliotibial band tightness, VMO hypoplasia, and foot biomechanics
- Contributing extrinsic factors include inappropriate or overly worn foot wear, precipitous changes in training volume, and poor training technique to name a few
- Symptoms arise from patellar chondral injury (chondromalacia patellae), synovial pinch, or synovitis

**Sx:**

- Symptoms typically begin 30–60 days after changing activity
- Pain is usually retro or peripatellar without associated joint line tenderness
- Exacerbated by running, climbing stairs, or sitting with the knee flexed for extended periods of time
- Sub-patellar grinding sensation and snapping or popping with activity are common
- Swelling is usually minimal
- Pain-related instability ("giving way") may occur

**Si:**

- Peripatellar tenderness, mild swelling, and small joint effusion
- Clinical signs of malalignment are common with a lateral "J" shift of the patella with active extension, increased "Q" angle, positive Ober's test (Fig. 11.1), and overpronated gait
- Patellar grind: the patient lies supine with the knee flexed 10°, pressure is applied to the proximal patella or quadriceps tendon as the patient actively flexes the quadriceps; the test is considered positive if it produces pain

**DiffDx:** Patellar tendinitis (see 12.9), plica syndrome (see 12.10), meniscal tear (see 12.3), bursitis (prepatellar, pes anserine) (see 12.11, 12.12), DJD

**Crs:** Arises with new activity or change in training; untreated, will commonly result in inability to participate

**Xray:** Lateralization of patella on AP view; lateral patellar tilt on sunrise view

**Rx:**

- Treatment goals are two-fold; symptom relief and rehabilitative exercises to improve functional patellar alignment
- PRICEMM (see 1.1) provides a useful guide for symptom modifying measures
- Patient should be educated regarding the etiology and contributing factors
- An aggressive physical therapy program should include quadriceps, IT band, and hamstring stretching, and balanced quadriceps strengthening (with particular attention to VMO strengthening)
- Typically, 30–60 days are required with specific limitations to running, jumping, and squatting activities
- The use of an open patella knee sleeve may also be helpful for symptom relief

- The patient should be instructed on alternative activities, such as cycling, swimming, or ski machine; should be prescribed during rehabilitation
- Occasionally, surgery may be useful in individuals with the more severe form (chondromalacia patellae); patients with severe symptoms and clinical evidence of chondromalacia should be referred for further evaluation

**Return to Activity:** As symptoms allow

# 12.9 TENDINITIS—PATELLAR OR QUADRICEPS

Am J Knee Surg 1999;12:99

**Cause:**
- Precipitated by excessive jumping or running with similar underlying intrinsic and extrinsic factors as found in RPPS (malalignment, poor shoe wear, technical deficiencies)
- Due to the association with these activities, this injury is often referred to as jumper's knee

**Epidem:** Most common in repetitive eccentric overload sports including basketball, volleyball, alpine skiing

**Pathophys:**
- Symptoms are due to inflammation of the tendon, usually at the insertion on the inferior pole of the patella
- Precipitated by eccentric overload

**Sx:**
- Anterior knee pain localized to the patellar or quadriceps tendon
- Mild swelling, erythema, and warmth
- Stiffness common after rest

**Si:**
- Examination reveals tenderness and soft tissue swelling along the patellar tendon particularly at the inferior pole of the patella
- Malalignment is typically seen with an increased Q angle, lateral patellar tracking, and weak ankle dorsiflexors
- The posterior muscle/tendon chain and the quadriceps tendon are generally tight

**Cmplc:**
- Predisposition to tendon rupture

**DiffDx:** RPPS (see 12.8), plica syndrome (see 12.10), meniscal tear (see 12.3), bursitis (prepatellar, pes anserine) (see 12.11, 12.12), DJD

**Crs:** Frequently results in chronic pain; can contribute to patellar tendon rupture if untreated

**Xray:** Lateralization of patella on AP view; lateral patellar tilt on sunrise view

**Rx:**
- Directed towards symptom relief initially with activity modification, NSAIDs, ice, and elevation
- Definitive therapy aims at correcting the functional malalignment and tightness through structured physical therapy
- The patient should be advised to continue in alternative, non-painful, activities while in rehabilitation
- The infrapatellar strap has been advocated for symptom relief and may be useful in some individuals

**Return to Activity:** As symptoms allow

## 12.10 MEDIAL PLICA SYNDROME

Am J Sports Med 1994;22:692

**Cause:** The plica may become inflamed either by a direct blow or through repetitive extension/flexion activities

**Epidem:** Synovial plica present in 20–60% of athletes

**Pathophys:**
- The synovial plica is an embryologic remnant that arises at the medial lining of the suprapatellar pouch and attaches to the synovium beneath the infrapatellar fat pad
- The medial edge of the plica protrudes from the medial joint in 20–50% of individuals

**Sx:** Chronic anteromedial knee pain which is worse with running or jumping activities

**Si:**
- There may be mild soft tissue swelling
- The plica is usually palpable along the medial patellofemoral joint with the knee held in slight flexion and the tibia internally rotated

**DiffDx:** RPPS (see 12.8), tendinitis (see 12.9), meniscal tear (see 12.3), bursitis (prepatellar, pes anserine) (see 12.11, 12.12), DJD

**Crs:** Frequently arises from an acute traumatic event then persists through repetitive motion injury

**Xray:** May show malalignment issues (patellar lateralization and tilt)

**Rx:**
- Activity modification and PRICEMM for symptom management
- Flexibility exercises for the posterior chain and quadriceps group
- Modification of functional malalignment as outlined for RPPS should also be done if malalignment is present
- Anti-inflammatory steroid injection often helpful for symptom management; triamcinolone (20–40 mg) with 2 to 3 cc of lidocaine is injected using sterile technique into the plica and surrounding soft tissue; care must be taken not to inject anteriorly in the area of the patellar tendon

**Return to Activity:** As symptoms allow

## 12.11 PREPATELLAR BURSITIS (HOUSEMAID'S KNEE, COAL MINER'S KNEE)

Am Fam Phys 1996;53:2317

**Cause:** This is usually associated with trauma, either chronic, as with repetitive kneeling (housemaid's knee), or an acute injury, such as a blow to the knee

**Epidem:** The prepatellar bursa is one of the most common sites for septic bursitis

**Pathophys:** Swelling in the bursa between the patella and skin; may be infectious or inflammatory

**Sx:** Anterior knee pain, stiffness, pain with motion; systemic signs of infection: fevers, chills, malaise

**Si:**
- Swelling anterior to the patella
- Infection should be considered if there is evidence of injury to the skin overlying the bursa
- Other frequent findings with infectious bursitis include increased warmth, redness, severe tenderness, lymphadenitis, cellulitis, and fever

**DiffDx:** RPPS (see 12.8), patellar tendinitis (see 12.9), plica syndrome (see 12.10)

**Crs:** Infectious bursitis may involve intra-articular knee if untreated

**Xray:** Negative

**Rx:**

- Aspiration should always be done if there is suspicion of an infection; this is done by first anesthetizing the skin with 1% lidocaine; a 22-gauge needle is inserted into the bursa under sterile conditions and the contents of the bursa aspirated using a 30 cc syringe
- The aspirate should be sent for analysis including: appearance, cell count, Gram stain, culture, and microscopy; approximately 90% of these infections are due to *Staphylococcus aureus* or *S. epidermidis* and 9% to streptococcal species; infectious bursitis requires drainage followed by antibiotic therapy
- Pending culture results, penicillinase resistant synthetic penicillins (dicloxacillin 500 mg qid), or first-generation cephalosporin (cephradine 500 mg qid) should be started
- In nonseptic cases, treatment follows the general outline described previously
- Wrapping the knee with an elastic bandage or padding for protection against further injury is helpful

**Return to Activity:** As symptoms allow

## 12.12 PES ANSERINE BURSITIS

Am Fam Phys 1996;53:2317

**Cause:** Direct blow to bursa or repetitive use of medial hamstring

**Epidem:** Most common in collision sports and in older athletes with DJD of knee

**Pathophys:** The pes anserine bursa lies behind the medial hamstring [formed by the tendons of the sartorius, gracilis and semitendinosus (SGT) muscles]

**Sx:** Pain and tenderness over the anteromedial aspect of the proximal tibia, 4–5 cm below the joint line that is exacerbated by active flexion of the knee

**Si:**

- Examination reveals swelling over the anteromedial tibia just proximal to the insertion of the SGT tendons which can be mistaken for a cyst or mass
- The tenderness may track along the SGT tendons indicating an associated tendinitis
- There is often evidence of patellar malalignment, as well as poor flexibility, particularly in the hamstrings and quadriceps tendons

**Crs:** Often chronic pain if untreated

**Xray:** Typically negative

**Rx:**

- Treatment follows the general PRICEMM guidelines
- Injected corticosteroids are very useful, however care must be taken not to inject the SGT tendons
- Particular attention should be given to stretching the hamstrings, quadriceps, and Achilles tendons

**Return to Activity:** As symptoms allow

## 12.13 POPLITEAL (BAKER'S) CYSTS

Am Fam Phys 1996;53:2317

**Cause:** Posterior knee swelling related to intra-articular effusion

**Epidem:** Seen most commonly in association with chronic meniscal disease or degenerative joint disease

**Pathophys:**

- Popliteal (Baker's) cysts usually arise from an intra-articular effusion
- Swelling of the medial gastrocnemius or semimembranosus bursae may also cause a painful popliteal cyst
- Popliteal cysts usually result from a significant intra-articular knee injury, osteoarthritis, rheumatoid arthritis, and less commonly, gouty arthritis

**Sx:** Symptoms include painful local swelling or popliteal mass that worsens with walking, jumping, or squatting

**Si:**

- Physical exam will usually demonstrate a tender mass in the popliteal fossa
- A careful examination of the knee must be done to rule out an associated internal derangement

**DiffDx:** Hamstring or popliteal tendinitis, meniscal tear (see 12.3), internal derangement

**Crs:** Chronic intermittent posterior knee pain

**Xray:**

- Plain radiographs may demonstrate degenerative joint disease
- Ultrasound or MRI are useful to differentiate an isolated semimembranosus bursa that communicates with the joint from a synovial hernia related to intra-articular pathology

**Rx:**

- Treatment in adults will often require surgery to correct intra-articular injury or to remove the cyst
- In children, popliteal cysts are usually not associated with intra-articular pathology and may be treated through observation after the diagnosis is confirmed by imaging studies
- Intra-articular corticosteroid injection is often effective to alleviate swelling and symptoms temporarily (see 2.13)

**Return to Activity:** As symptoms allow

## 12.14 ILIOTIBIAL BAND FRICTION SYNDROME (ITBFS)

Med Sci Sports Exerc 1995;27:951

**Cause:** Tightness in the ITB leads to friction irritation at the lateral femoral condyle resulting in inflammation and pain

**Epidem:** Common in runners, dancers, and cross-country skiers

**Pathophys:**

- The iliotibial band (ITB) arises from the tensor fascia lata muscle in the lateral buttocks and runs along the lateral leg to its insertion at Gerdy's tubercle on the anteriolateral tibia
- Predisposing factors include genu varum, leg length discrepancy, excessive foot pronation, as well as running on sloped surfaces such as the cambered surface of a road

**Sx:**

- These patients complain of lateral knee pain that is worse with activities such as running, jumping, and squatting
- Character of pain frequently described as aching

**Si:**

- Marked tenderness and swelling along the distal course of the ITB as it crosses the femoral condyle
- Ober's sign: the patient is placed on their side and both hips flexed 90° with the knees flexed to 90°, the free leg is then maximally extended; tightness in the ITB is demonstrated if the knee does not fall to the table (Fig. 11.1)

**DiffDx:** Lateral meniscal tear (see 12.3), lateral collateral ligament tear (see 12.7)

**Crs:** Acute irritation often becomes chronic pain if left untreated.

**Xray:** Xray negative; MRI may demonstrate effusion between ITB and lat femoral condyle

**Rx:**

- Pain relief and anti-inflammatory measures follow the general guidelines of PRICEMM (see 1.1)
- Corticosteroid injection (triamcinolone 40 mg, or betamethasone 6 mg) is useful for symptom relief; the tender area is identified (usually at the lateral femoral condyle), the steroid is injected beneath the ITB under sterile technique; typically 2 to 3 cc of lidocaine is mixed with the steroid to provide immediate relief
- Physical therapy is directed at improving ITB flexibility through stretching exercise
- Treatment should also address any foot biomechanical issues and underlying sacroiliac dysfunction

**Return to Activity:** As symptoms allow

# 13 Leg Problems

## 13.1 STRESS FRACTURES

Clin Sport Med 1997;16:259; Med Sci Sport Ex 2000;32:S15

**Cause:** Increase in running mileage, intensity, change in training shoes or poor training shoes, change to a harder or different running surface; most commonly occur in the tibia (Am J Sports Med 1987;15:46)

**Epidem:** Runners, sports involving running, military recruits; incidence higher in women, especially in women with irregular menses

**Pathophys:**
- Imbalance between bone resorption and bone deposition during host bone response to stress
- Microfractures progress to clinical stress fractures in the setting of continuing abusive activity and inadequate rest

**Sx:** Pain, commonly in the proximal anterior tibia; initially present after activity, progressing to pain during activity, then pain preventing activity; if pain is in the distal lateral aspect of leg, a fibular stress fracture may be present (see Chapter 14); swelling may accompany stress fractures

**Si:** Tenderness over the tibia or fibula, localized to an area less than 5 cm in diameter, is very suggestive of a stress fracture

**Cmplc:** Progression to complete fracture, nonunion of fracture, displacement of fracture, chronic disabling leg pain; athletes with stress fracture in the anterior central third of the tibia are very slow to heal and have a high risk of progression to complete fracture

**DiffDx:** MTSS (see 13.4), tibialis posterior syndrome, exertional compartment syndrome (see 13.2), fascial hernia, tumor

**Xray:**

- AP and lateral radiographs may show stress fractures that have been symptomatic for more than 3 weeks; beware the anterior cortical tibial dreaded black line ("DBL")
- Focal periosteal thickening may be seen, actual fracture line is rare
- Bone scan will be positive 3–5 days after the onset of pain

**Rx:** Stop pain-producing activities (including weight bearing if injury has progressed); healing time is 4–6 weeks for noncomplicated stress fractures; if able to perform pain-free, cycling or swimming may be done to maintain fitness

**Return to Activity:** Should be gradual; use of pneumatic leg braces has been shown in a small study to reduce healing time by up to several week (Am J Sports Med 1987;15:86)

## 13.2 EXERTIONAL COMPARTMENT SYNDROME (ECS)

Orthop Rev 1994;23:219; Med Sci Sport Ex 2000;32(3):S4

**Cause:** Overuse injury in runners from impact activities

**Epidem:** Runners, athletes in sports requiring running

**Pathophys:**

- Exercise induced soft tissue swelling in the limited volume of the fascial compartments produces ischemia
- The compartments most frequently affected by ECS are the anterior, followed by the deep posterior, lateral, posterior tibial, and superficial posterior

**Table 13–1. Four Fascial Compartments of the Leg**

| Compartment | Muscles | Nerve | Sensory Area |
|---|---|---|---|
| Lateral | Peroneus brevis and longus | Superficial peroneal nerve | Dorsal foot |
| Anterior | Tibialis ant, ext digitorum, and hallucis | Deep peroneal nerve | Dorsal first web space |
| Deep posterior | Flexor digit/hallux, posterior tibialis | Tibial nerve | Plantar foot |
| Superficial posterior | Soleus, gastrocnemius | Sural foot | Lateral foot |

**Sx:**

- Exercise-induced aching, squeezing or sharp pain in the anterior leg, relieved by rest
- May be bilateral
- Pain often recurs at the same distance while running
- May have muscle or nerve dysfunction in the affected compartment
- Anterior leg may be diffusely swollen and described as "tense" (Sports Injuries, Diagnosis and Management. Philadelphia: Saunders Company; 1999, p 350)

**Si:**

- Tenderness over the involved compartment
- Fascial herniae are present in up to 46% of cases
- Neurovascular exam is commonly normal, however, paresthesia may be present in affected legs; if the anterior compartment is affected, slight foot drop may be present as well as decreased sensation in the first web space of the foot
- Diagnosis is confirmed by measuring pre-exercise and post-exercise intracompartmental pressures; the necessary equipment is currently available in kit form
- The American Academy of Orthopaedic Surgeons have published the following diagnostic standards:
    1. Resting pressure exceeding 15 mm Hg before exercise
    2. 1-min post-exercise pressure exceeding 30 mm Hg

**Cmplc:** Chronic leg pain; progression of neurovascular deficit

**DiffDx:** MTSS (see 13.4), stress fracture (see 13.1)

**Xray:** R/o stress fx; consider bone scan in refractory cases

**Rx:**

- Nonoperative treatment is cessation or reduction of running (or aggravating activity)
- Cross training may be attempted
- Operative treatment consists of fasciotomy of all affected compartments, with good overall results and return to full activity at 1-month post surgery

## 13.3 TENNIS LEG

Ankle 1985;5:186

**Cause:** Partial or total rupture of the medial head of the gastrocnemius muscle

**Epidem:** Common muscle injury in men older than 40 years participating in racquet sports, alpine skiing, and running; occurs twice as frequently in men

**Pathophys:** Partial tear at the musculotendinous junction of the medial belly of the gastrocnemius muscle; injury occurs with the knee fully extended and the ankle maximally dorsiflexed

**Sx:** Sudden sharp pain in mid posteromedial leg leading to an obligate immediate stop of sport activity; may report feeling that the back of the leg was hit, may hear or feel a "pop"; intense pain with walking

**Si:** Tenderness with local pressure or stretching; local defect can be palpated for a few hours post-injury; substantial swelling immediately and ecchymosis within 1–2 days

**Cmplc:** Deep-vein thrombosis secondary to extrinsic compression and immobilization; compartment syndrome

**DiffDx:** Deep-vein thrombosis (Clin Sports Med 1997;16:475)

**Xray:** Ultrasonography is able to demonstrate the size of the lesion

**Rx:**
- Rest, ice, elevation for the first 48 hours, with crutches for ambulating
- Short use of a ROM or CAM walker for immobilization in more severe cases
- Neoprene sleeve for muscle support
- Passive then active stretching of calf by 2 weeks
- Heal pad may make walking more comfortable until calf is able to stretch

**Return to Activity:** Gradual return to activity when walking pain free; recovery time generally 4–12 weeks

## 13.4 MEDIAL TIBIAL STRESS SYNDROME (MTSS OR SHIN SPLINTS)

Am J Sports Med 1985;13:398; Med Sci Sport Ex 2000;32:S27

**Cause:** Overuse injury cause by running by a deconditioned athlete or sudden increase in intensity of training

**Epidem:** Runners, jumpers, and participants in sports requiring running

**Pathophys:**
- Has been attributed to stress along medial fascial insertion of the soleus muscle (soleus bridge) causing myositis, fasciitis, and periostitis
- Some have implicated the posterior tibialis
- Excessive foot pronation has been implicated; the athlete is forced to pronate to accommodate for gastro-soleus inflexibility

**Sx:**
- Pain along the posterior medial border of the distal tibia, induced by exercise and relieved by rest
- Initially pain is after activity
- Pain at the start of activity, relieved during activity, and returning after activity is consistent with MTSS
- Pain with resisted plantar flexion and inversion

**Si:** Exquisite tenderness along the posterior medial border of the distal third to the tibia; pain with standing on toes; pronated feet are a common finding

**Cmplc:** Chronic leg pain and poor performance

**DiffDx:** Exertional compartment syndrome of the deep posterior compartment (see 13.2); stress fracture (see 13.1); tumor

**Xray:**
- Radiographs normal
- Longitudinally oriented diffuse uptake involving $1/3$ or more of the length of the bone are present on bone scan

**Rx:**
- Rest for 1 week, with a very gradual return to full activity
- Excessive pronators will benefit from fitted orthotics
- Gastroc-soleus stretching
- Other modalities, including NSAIDs, icing, crutches, steriods, etc., have not been shown to decrease healing time over rest alone

# 14 Ankle Injuries

## Acute Injuries

### 14.1 LATERAL ANKLE SPRAIN

Clin Sports Med 1997;16:433; Phy Sportsmed 1993;21(3):123; Phy
   Sportsmed 1998;26(10):29

**Cause:** Excessive, rapid ankle inversion; the majority of ankle sprains
   involve the anterior talofibular ligament

**Epidem:** Most common injury in athletics; 85% of all ankle injuries are
   sprains; 85% are lateral, and 85% involve the anterior talofibular
   ligaments (ATFL)

**Pathophys:** Inversion or an internal rotation force to a plantar-flexed
   ankle, which may result in partial or complete disruption of the
   lateral ligamentous complex (ATFL), calcaneofibular (CFL), and,
   much less commonly, the posterior talofibular ligaments (PTFL)

**Sx:** The patient may appreciate a "tear" or "pop" at the time of injury,
   which may indicate a complete tear; the pain is intense and
   localized to the lateral ankle; the pain may initially improve in the
   first few hours, only to return with the presence of increased
   swelling; normal ROM is dorsiflexion (DF) 15° to 20°, plantar
   flexion (PF) 50°, eversion (Ev), inversion (Inv)

**Si:**
   • Tenderness to palpation (TTP) with or without swelling over ATFL,
     CFL, or PTFL
   • Ecchymosis over lateral ankle
   • Decreased active ROM
   • Assess sensation in the distribution of the deep peroneal nerve
     (first webbed space of the foot)
   • Assess motor function and presence of dorsalis pedis and posterior
     tibial pulses

- May have positive talar tilt test

    Performed with the patient seated and with the ankle in 10° of plantar flexion

    Stabilize the medial aspect of the distal part of the leg just proximal to the medial malleolus with one hand and apply an inversion force slowly to the hindfoot with the other hand; the affected side is compared against the normal side; if the talus gaps and rocks open, this indicates laxity of the ATFL

- May have positive anterior drawer test

    Performed with the foot in 10° of plantar flexion: tests for anterolateral rotatory instability due to anterior talofibular ligament instability

    Stabilize the distal part of the leg with one hand and apply an anterior force with the other hand on the heel; attempt to subluxate the talus anteriorly from beneath the tibia (Fig. 14.1)

    The affected ankle is compared to the patient's normal ankle

    Alternative anterior drawer test may be performed by having the patient rest each foot on the examining table with the knees bent @ 90 degrees; the examiner then stabilizes the foot on the exam table and provides a posterior force on the distal tibia and estimates the degree of posterior diplacement of the tibia on the talus (anterior drawer)

- Talar tilt and anterior drawer tests may be difficult to perform in acute setting

*Grading sprains:*

- Grade I: mild stretching of the fibers within the ligament but produce no evidence of laxity; disability 1–2 wks
- Grade II: partial tear of ATFL and CFL with mild laxity but good overall stability; disability 2–4 wks
- Grade III: complete rupture of ATFL and CFL and cause unstable joint associated with peroneal nerve damage; disability 2 to 6 months.

**Cmplc:** Traction injuries of the peroneal and posterior tibial nerves can occur in severe injuries; peroneal compartment syndrome; chronic

**DiffDx:** Syndesmotic injury (see 14.3), peroneal tendon subluxation (see 14.2), talar dome lesion (see 14.4), ankle fracture, Achilles tendon rupture (see 14.5), mid-foot injury (see 15.14), lateral process fracture of the talus (prevalent in snow boarders, poorly visible on x-ray, CT if suspect)

**ANKLE INJURIES**

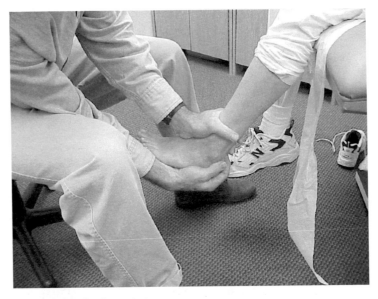

**Figure 14.1.** Anterior drawer test

**Xray:**
- To rule out fracture or syndesmotic injury
- Standard: AP, lateral, and mortise views
- Consider foot and leg films when clinically indicated
- The radiographs should be evaluated for:
  1. The presence or absence of a medial malleolar fracture or widening of the space between the medial malleolus and the talus
  2. The presence or absence of a fibular fracture, its relationship to the tibial plafond (i.e., at, above, or below), and the orientation of the fracture (i.e., transverse, oblique, or comminuted)
  3. Displacement of the distal tibiofibular joint (to assess competency of the syndesmosis)
  4. Displacement of the talus from its normal anatomic position beneath the tibia
- Ottawa rules: a decision protocol designed to avoid obtaining films on all ankle injuries by identifying patients at negligible risk for

fracture; Ottawa rules have a 97%+ sensitivity for ruling out a fracture, but only a 31–63% specificity for ruling in fractures (JAMA 1993;269:1127), essentially an ankle x-ray series is necessary only if there is pain near the malleoli and any of these findings:

Inability to bear weight both immediately and in the emergency room (four steps), or

Bone tenderness at the posterior edge or tip of either malleolus

- Radiographic assessment of the syndesmosis: one of the more challenging and important tasks that the clinician must perform is to rule out an injury to the syndesmosis; the mortise and AP views must be utilized to review the criteria for diagnosing injury to the syndesmosis

Rx: Refer to orthopedic surgeon if medial clear space is greater than 2 mm greater than superior, all medial malleolar fractures, and lateral malleolar fracture with over 2 mm displacement; early protected mobilization and functional rehabilitation for all grades of sprain; ankle rehabilitation (modified from Physical Therapy Department, U.S. Naval Academy)

*Phase I:* (Immediate postinjury) **PRICEMM and early motion**

- Use crutches or cane if unable to walk without limp; emphasize normal heel–toe gait with progressive weight bearing over 1–5 d
- PRICEMM

**P**rotect from further damage: ankle brace to limit inversion and eversion

**R**elative rest: limit activity; avoid abusing activity

**I**ce: apply for 20 min at least 3–4 times per d

**C**ompression: wrap ankle with ace wrap or ankle brace to control swelling; horse-shoe felt around lateral malleolus may improve effectiveness of compression wraps

**E**levate: keep leg above the heart as much as possible to help control swelling

**M**edications: large scale studies have demonstrated that nonsteroidal anti-inflammatory drug (NSAID) used postinjury resulted in reduced subject pain, time lost from training, cost of treatment, and increased exercise endurance; however, NSAID use was also associated with increased ligament laxity, decreased ROM, and increased swelling; it is possible that the analgesic effects allow athletes to resume training prematurely (Am I Sports Med 1997;25:544); if NSAIDs are used, consider starting 48 hrs postinjury to decrease risk of increased bleeding at injury site; acetaminophen for pain as needed

Modalities: Physical therapy (e-stim or ultrasound)

- Ice bath followed by stationary bike: immerse foot in ice bucket until foot is numb, and then ride bike until numbness wears off; repeat 4 times
- ROM exercise: write the capital letters of the alphabet with the big toe by moving at the ankle; only move to the point of stretching

*Phase II*: Begin as soon as one can tolerate the listed activity without compensation

- Stationary bike
- Range-of-motion exercise (DF, PF, eversion, inversion)
- Balance and proprioception exercises: BAPS, foam roller balance
- Theraband exercises: loop theraband or surgical tubing around forefoot, hold proximal ends in hands; invert and evert against resistance
- Heel raises and Achilles stretching: raise up on the balls of both feet, lifting the heels off the floor; lower the heels slowly; 30 repetitions; when stronger, raise up on strong foot, lower with only the injured foot
- Contrast bath: 20 min

*Phase III*: Begin when able to walk without limp

- Add stairmaster, slide board, squats, and lunges
- Balance and proprioception exercises: stand on affected leg on minitrampoline; close eyes for 20 sec (go ahead and try it while you're healthy—it is an ankle workout); repeat 6 times; stand on affected leg on minitrampoline, play catch with someone with a 1–2 kilogram medicine ball (or any ball)
- Ice ankle after exercise for 20 min

*Phase IV*:

- Gradual return to jogging
- Jump rope
- Dot jumping, agility drills, balance and proprioception exercises
- Ice as needed
- Consider ankle brace for return to full activity
- Progression from phase to phase is dependent upon individual progression, NOT time

*Prevention*: Most common risk factor for ankle sprain is a history of previous sprain; supervised rehabilitation should be complete before return to practice; athletes suffering a moderate or severe sprain should wear an appropriate brace for at least 6 months; properly fitting braces or correctly applied tape does not interfere with athletic performance; ankle taping provides effective support for less than 20 min of exercise, however it may help provide additional proprioception via the skin and reduce injury, lace-up braces and stirrup-style braces offer longer lasting support; ankle strengthening and proprioception training (see Phase IV of ankle rehabilitation) are the most effective form of prevention (Am J Sports Med 1999;277:573)

**Return to Activity:**
- Normal range of motion
- 85% of pre-injury strength
- Minimal swelling
- No pain with ADLs
- Pain-free execution of functional drills such as hopping on injured leg or sprinting tight figure eight pattern
- Good proprioception as demonstrated by ability to single leg stand with eyes closed for 25–30 sec

# 14.2 PERONEAL TENDON SUBLUXATION AND DISLOCATION

Handbook of Sports Medicine: A Symptom-Oriented Approach, 2nd ed. Boston: Butterworth and Heinemann, 1999; p 287

**Cause:** Acute dorsiflexion and inversion stress to the ankle

**Epidem:** Thus injury is associated with a wide variety of sporting activity, most commonly in skiing (71%), football (7%), and basketball

**Pathophys:** Sudden and forceful inversion and dorsiflexion of foot result in rupture of inferior or superior retinaculum, which normally channel the peroneal tendon; it often occurs in conjunction with anterolateral ankle instability

**Sx:** The athlete generally notes a "pop" and/or snapping sensation posterior to the lateral malleolus

**Si:** Tenderness posterior and inferior to lateral malleolus; palpable subluxation of the tendon with active dorsiflexion and eversion against resistance

**Cmplc:** Often misdiagnosed as lateral sprain; nonoperative treatment may lead to chronic lateral ankle pain and instability

**Xray:** Radiographs may reveal a fracture-avulsion of the lateral ridge of the fibula

**Rx:**
- Treatment in the active individual is controversial
- Results with closed treatment are generally disappointing
- Consider early referral to orthopedics

## 14.3 SYNDESMOSIS INJURY (HIGH ANKLE SPRAIN)

Phys Sports Med 1993;21:39

**Cause:** Ankle pronation with abduction or external or internal rotation

**Epidem:** Football and wrestling

**Pathophys:** Injury to the syndesmotic ligaments of the ankle; the syndesmotic ligaments consist of the anterior inferior tibiofibular ligament (AITFL), the posterior inferior tibiofibular ligament (PITFL), and the interosseous ligament (IOM) (primary bond between the tibia and fibula); can result in diastasis between the tibia and fibula at the ankle

**Sx:** Can appear benign initially; pain along the interosseous membrane, pain proximal and anterior on the ankle; isolated injury to the syndesmosis without fracture not common, and often associated with medial ankle sprain; athlete presents with marked discomfort and swelling: often unable to bear weight

**Si:** Often there is minimal swelling, especially in isolated injuries

*Positive Squeeze Test:* Apply compression with one or two hands to the midpoint of the calf; the test is positive if compression produces pain at distal tib–fib

*Positive Cotton Test (External Rotation Test):*
- Stabilize the distal lower leg with one hand while grasping each side of the foot at the talus with the thumb and forefinger of the other hand (Fig. 14.2)
- Apply a mediolateral force (externally rotate the foot) and assess crepitus, instability, or pain
- Increased motion or pain in the anterior tib–fib area or anywhere along the fibula is a positive test

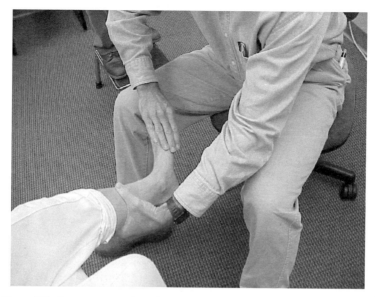

**Figure 14.2.** Cotton or external rotation test for syndesmotic pain

**Cmplc:** Maisonneuve's fracture is syndesmosis sprain with fracture, typically involves complete rupture of the deltoid ligament, the ATFL, and IOM and a proximal fibula fracture; failure to recognize radiographic evidence of syndesomosis injury results in prolonged disability; bony avulsions from tibia.

**DiffDx:** Ankle sprain (see 14.1), OCD of the talar dome (see 14.4), loose body, instability

**Xray:** Mortise view to assess mortise alignment of tibia, talus, and fibula; weight bearing views recommended

- Mortise view abnormal if:
    The tibiofibular clear space is greater than 6 mm on AP and mortise views
    There is less than 6 mm of overlap of the tibia and fibula at the incisura fibularis on AP view
    Less than 1 mm of tibia and fibula overlap on the mortise view
- Use comparison with uninjured ankle if unclear; AP and lateral of lower leg to rule out Maisonneuve's fracture

**Rx:**
- For ankle sprain without fracture and without radiographic evidence of syndesmotic injury, standard ankle rehabilitation; recovery time 9 weeks +
- For injuries with radiographic evidence of syndesmotic injury, with or without associated fracture, refer to orthopedic surgeon for stabilization with syndesmosis screw

## 14.4 OSTEOCHONDRAL DEFECT OF THE TALUS (OCD)

Phys Sports Med 1993;21(3):109

**Cause:** Traumatic or idiopathic etiologies

**Epidem:** Osteochondral injuries/fractures not uncommonly occur in association with inversion ankle sprain; these tibio–talar intra-articular fractures occur when there is a compressive component involved in the mechanism of injury; the fractures most commonly involve the anterolateral and posteromedial aspects of the talus; OCL typically appears in the younger athlete

**Pathophys:** Forceful inversion of the dorsiflexed ankle results in an intra-articular anterolateral lesion; posteromedial lesions result from inversion of the plantar-flexed ankle

**Sx:**
- Athletes describe pain "inside" their ankle
- These injuries are frequently missed on initial examination and it is only when the patient presents with prolonged pain or aching, persistent swelling, and/or perhaps catching, locking, or giving way, that the diagnosis is contemplated
- Activity related swelling

**Si:**
- The patient may have tenderness over the dome of the talus
- Tenderness to palpation over anterolateral or posteromedial aspect of ankle
- Palpable lesion, detectable with posterior lesion in maximum plantar flexion, effusion, decreased range of motion, pain with inversion or eversion, and crepitus may be present
- Exam may be normal

**Cmplc:** Chronic ankle pain, accelerated OA, mechanical symptoms (locking) from loose body

**DiffDx:** OA, anterolateral soft tissue impingement (see 14.7), instability, poorly rehabilitated lateral ankle sprain (see 14.1)

**Xray:**

- Findings often subtle, radiographs (plantar flexion views) may demonstrate a discrete fragment in an acute injury and subchondral sclerosis and/or cysts in the subacute or chronic presentation
- If plain films are normal, and the diagnostic suspicion is high, a bone scan with coned down views of foot and ankle should be ordered
- A positive bone scan warrants further evaluation with a high resolution CT or MRI

**Rx:** Refer for appropriate staging and management; treatment may range from a nonweight-bearing cast to open reduction and internal fixation

## 14.5 ACHILLES TENDON RUPTURE

Am J Sports Med 1993;21:791

**Cause:** Occurs after a sudden dorsiflexion of a plantar flexed foot; eccentric load from a cutting motion or sudden change of direction on a court

**Epidem:** Not uncommonly seen in athletes in the 4th and 5th decades of life; common in basketball, base running in baseball, or court sports

**Pathophys:** Rupture or partial rupture of Achilles tendon; relative avascular zone 6 cm proximal to insertion

**Sx:** The athlete may complain of a sudden "pop" in the heel or reports a feeling of being shot or kicked in the heel, followed by difficulty walking

**Si:**

- May have a palpable defect in the tendon 2–3 cm proximal to the heel
- Positive Thompson test (Fig. 14.3)

    Patient lies prone on the examining table with the feet extending over the end of the exam table

    The examiner squeezes the middle third of the gastroc-soleus and observes for movement of the dorsiflexed foot into a position of plantar flexion

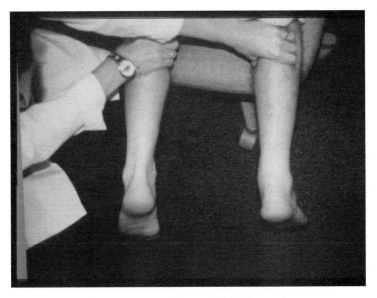

**Figure 14.3.** Thompson squeeze test (left normal; right abnormal)

The test can also be performed with the patient kneeling on a chair

Absence of plantar flexion suggests a disruption of the Achilles tendon

**Cmplc:** Failure to promptly diagnose may limit operative repair and prolong disability; ankle sprain is the most common initial misdiagnosis

**DiffDx:** Gastroc or soleus strain (see 13.3), Achilles tendinopathy (see 14.11), retrocalcaneal bursitis (see 15.17)

**Xray:** If necessary MRI can establish a definitive diagnosis

**Rx:**

• Initial management: posterior, nonweight bearing splint with 45° plantar flexion; crutches, ice, pain medications, elevation

• Refer for operative repair, which has been demonstrated to provide superior strength, endurance, and a lower risk of re-rupture in the athlete

- If nonoperative treatment is elected, cast in gravity equinus position (gravity induced plantar flexion) in long or short leg cast; no weight bearing on leg for 8 weeks, crutches for mobility; consider recasting in reduced plantar flexion at 4 weeks; after 8 weeks, the cast is removed and a 2.5-cm heel lift is worn for 4 weeks

## 14.6 POSTERIOR TIBIALIS TENDON RUPTURE

Handbook of Sports Medicine: A Symptom-Oriented Approach, 2nd ed. Boston: Butterworth, 1999; p 283

**Cause:** Sudden plantar flexion, usually preceded by chronic medial ankle pain and associated with aging

**Epidem:** Common clinical entity seen in mature female athletes who engage in hiking and patients with hyper-mobile flat feet; also seen in sports requiring quick changes in direction (e.g., soccer and basketball)

**Pathophys:** The repetitive microtrauma of excessive pronation is thought to result in degenerative changes in tendon leading to acute disruption

**Sx:** Difficulty walking with or without pain and swelling immediately posterior to the medial malleolus; pain is worse with ambulation; rarely associated with trauma

**Si:**
- Classically, the patient presents with *unilateral fallen arch* when standing
- When viewed from behind, the patient demonstrates the "too many toes" sign on the lateral aspect of the affected foot secondary to abduction of the forefoot
- When the patient is asked to stand on his or her toes, the affected foot is unable to demonstrate the normal inversion secondary to an absent posterior tibialis
- Soft tissue swelling posterior to the medial malleolus; the pain is aggravated by inversion and plantar flexion against resistance

**Cmplc:** Potential for severe disability

**Xray:** In cases where the diagnosis is unclear, MRI is the test of choice

**Rx:** Refer for operative repair

# Chronic Injuries

## 14.7 ANTEROLATERAL SOFT-TISSUE IMPINGEMENT

Am J Sports Med 1998;253:89

**Cause:** Anterolateral impingement of the ankle soft tissues secondary to repeated ankle sprains

**Epidem:** Activities such as gymnastics, tennis, soccer, football, and ballet have been commonly noted to result in anterior tibiotalar impingement; often seen in athlete whose ankle is not aggressively rehabilitated after previous sprain

**Pathophys:** The dome of the talus rubs against the hypertrophied and scarred anterior inferior tibiofibular ligament, causing reactive tissue formation; repeated injury can result in synovial hypertrophy and/or a meniscoid lesion that is commonly identified in the anterolateral gutter

**Sx:** Chronic persistent anterior ankle pain, intermittent catching, and/or swelling; generally worse with activity; occasionally, a popping or snapping sensation with dorsiflexion; pain with walking uphill

**Si:** The most ratable clinical finding is restriction and painful dorsiflexion of the ankle; tenderness to palpation over the anterior talocrural joint

**Cmplc:** Progression to constant pain

**DiffDx:** Loose body, OCD (see 14.4), OA, peroneal tendon tendinopathy or subluxation (see 14.2)

**Xray:** Exostoses are generally present on lateral radiographs; non-weight bearing lateral flexion and extension views will demonstrate the impingement; plain films may be normal

**Rx:**
- Aggressive Achilles stretching program, relative rest, and modification of activity (e.g., no hill running)
- Ice and contrast baths to affected area
- Diagnosis may be confirmed with single injection of the ATFL with 1 cc lidocaine
- If a good response to diagnostic injection, the provider may consider a follow-up injection with lidocaine and 6 mg Celestone or 20 mg Kenalog for treatment

- Failure of 4 weeks of conservative therapy should be referred for possible arthroscopic resection

## 14.8 POSTERIOR TIBIALIS TENDINOPATHY

The Lower Extremity and Spine in Sports Medicine, 2nd ed, St. Louis; Mosby; 1995; p 441

**Cause:** Degenerative changes in tendon associated with aging

**Epidem:** Common clinical entity seen in mature female athletes who engage in hiking and patients with hypermobile flat feet; also seen in sports requiring quick changes in direction (e.g., soccer and basketball)

**Pathophys:** The repetitive microtrauma of excessive pronation is thought to result in degenerative changes in tendon leading to acute disruption

**Sx:** Difficulty walking; pain and swelling immediately posterior to the medial malleolus; the pain is worse when bearing weight and ambulating; rarely associated with trauma

**Si:** Tenderness to palpation immediately posterior to the medial malleolus, frequently associated crepitance; soft tissue swelling posterior to the medial malleolus; the pain is aggravated by inversion and plantar flexion against resistance

**Cmplc:** Rupture, tarsal tunnel syndrome, chronic pain and dysfunction

**DiffDx:** Tarsal tunnel syndrome (see 15.18), tarsal navicular stress fracture (see 15.11), deltoid ligament sprain

**Xray:** MRI may demonstrate degeneration

**Rx:**
- Rest, modification of abusive activities (including weight bearing if aggravating)
- Ice massage
- NSAIDs
- Foot orthosis to decrease pronation
- Slow toe raises, accentuating the lowering phase, should be started when able to do the exercise pain free
- In the young athlete with acute inflammation or in severe cases, immobilization in a short leg, nonweight bearing cast with the foot in slight inversion for 10 day often relieves the symptoms
- Refer refractory cases to consider tenodesis (surgical mangement)

## 14.9 SINUS TARSI SYNDROME

The Lower Extremity and Spine in Sports Medicine, 2nd ed. St. Louis: Mosby; 1995, p 437

**Cause:** Post-traumatic, force inversion of the foot

**Epidem:** History of multiple prior ankle sprains

**Pathophys:** The syndrome is generally secondary to a prolonged synovitis following a subtalar joint injury; one proposed factor in the pathogenesis is posttraumatic fibrotic changes in the tissue surrounding the veins draining the sinus, resulting in increased intrasinusal pressure (Clin Anat 1997;10:173)

**Sx:** Pain over the lateral opening of the sinus tarsi (talocalcaneal sulcus) along with a feeling of instability

**Si:** Tenderness over lateral side of the foot that is increased by firm pressure over the sinus tarsi and inversion of the foot; relief with 2–3 cc of lidocaine directly into the sinus tarsi confirms the diagnosis

**Cmplc:** Chronic pain

**DiffDx:** Anterolateral soft tissue impingement (see 14.7), lateral ankle sprain (see 14.1), bifurcate ligament injury, cuboid/talus/calcaneal stress fx (see 15.13), OA, OCD (see 14.4)

**Xray:** Radiographs are unremarkable

**Rx:** Treatment is difficult and should include complete ankle rehabilitation; relative rest, avoidance of aggravating activities and NSAIDs should be started; if unsuccessful, corticosteroid injection to the sinus tarsi may provide relief, multiple injections may be necessary; if conservative treatment fails, surgical debridement of the sinus tarsi can be helpful

## 14.10 DISTAL FIBULAR STRESS FRACTURE

Handbook of Sports Medicine: A Symptom-Oriented Approach, 2nd ed. Boston: Butterworth, 1999; p 27

**Cause:** History of overuse and activity related lateral ankle pain

**Epidem:** Runners

**Pathophys:** Chronic insult to distal fibula

**Sx:** On occasion, the athlete may note some mild swelling above the lateral ankle; the pain generally improves with rest; symptoms usually gradual in onset over a 2- to 3-week period

**Si:** Focal bony tenderness 2–7 cm proximal to the lateral malleolus

**Cmplc:** Complete fracture

**DiffDx:** Peroneal tendinopathy or strain (see 14.2), exertional compartment syndrome (see 13.2)

**Xray:** Radiographs frequently reveal a focal periosteal reaction; if negative, a bone scan is confirmatory

**Rx:** Stop abusive activity for a period of 4–6 weeks as the bone remodels; the athlete may participate in nonweight-bearing cross-training activities; upon return to sport, shock absorbing insoles and "forgiving" running surfaces may help; the most important preventive feature, however, is to avoid doing too much, too soon

## 14.11 ACHILLES TENDINOPATHY

Am J Sports Med 1998;26:360

**Cause:** Overuse, increase in mileage, increase in hill running, poor calf/hamstring flexibility

**Epidem:** Common injury in runners, athletes in their 30s and 40s

**Pathophys:**

- Degenerative changes in Achilles tendon from chronic insult (see 1.1)
- Histology of affected tendons reveal this condition (and other chronic over-use injuries) is not associated with inflammation, hence, the term tendinopathy instead of the most familiar tendinitis, which implies inflammation

**Sx:** Activity-related pain localized to the tendon, approximately 3–4 cm above its insertion into the calcaneus; recent change in shoes and/or training

**Si:** Tenderness and possibly focal swelling and/or crepitus in the tendon; in chronic tendinopathy, the tendon is often thickened and nodular; hamstring and gastroc-soleus inflexibility, as well as evidence of functional overpronation are common

**Cmplc:** Achilles tendon rupture (see 14.5), chronic pain and dysfunction

**DiffDx:** Peritendonitis, retrocalcaneal bursitis (see 15.17)

**Xray:** MRI of lower leg if confirmation is needed

**Rx:**

*Initial:* Relative rest from the offending activity (cross train); then modification of activities to include decreasing mileage and avoiding hill running; orthotics to correct pathologic over-pronation; heavy eccentric (stretching phase) exercise

- The healthy leg executes a toe raise, and the injured leg slowly lowers the body weight for 3 sets of 15 reps with the injured leg straight and 15 reps with the injured flexed 15 degrees
- Additional weight is added in a backpack as strength is gained
- Gentle slow calf stretching on slant board or block is performed least 3 times a day
- This routine is done daily for 3 months, with gradual return to running as tolerated during this time

Severe cases can be temporarily casted in the equinus (plantar flexed) position for 2–4 weeks, refer recalcitrant cases for surgical debridement

# 15  Foot Problems

## Skin and Nails

### 15.1 BLISTERS

Phy Sportsmed 1999;27(1):57; 1997;25(12):45
**Cause:** Repeated friction on the skin surface
**Epidem:** Common, potentially debilitating injury; often occur early in the season
**Pathophys:** Acute response to high intensity stress that produces a shear force that separates the skin into two layers; the space fills with fluid secondary to hemodynamic forces
**Sx:** Pain
**Si:** Vessicle that may be filled with blood or purulent fluid; tender to palpation
**Crs:** May rupture with persistent activity
**Cmplc:** May become infected
**Rx:**

- Prevention includes appropriately fitted shoes and socks, padding hot spots, lubricants
- Acute treatment includes possible drainage, use of a blister care product (Second Skin, Compeed), antibiotic ointment, and protective padding
- Care must be taken to keep the site clean to avoid infection

**FOOT PROBLEMS**

## 15.2 SUBUNGUAL HEMATOMA

The Foot and Ankle in Sport. St. Louis: Mosby; 1995, p 133; Primary
   Care Sports Medicine. Dubuque, IA: Brown & Benchmark; 1993,
   p 448; Phy Sportsmed 1999;27(9):35
**Cause:** Improperly fitted shoes; downhill running; direct trauma
**Epidem:** Common in long distance runners
**Pathophys:** Shearing or crushing injury in which there is bleeding under
   the toenail
**Sx:** Pain
**Si:** Blood under the nail; may be tender
**Crs:** Gradually resolves; the nail may fall off at some future point
**Cmplc:** Loss of the nail
**Xray:** Rule out fracture in cases of direct trauma
**Rx:**
   • Appropriately fitted shoes may prevent this problem
   • If hemorrhage is acute and painful, it can be relieved by drilling
     a hole in the nail, using a heated 18-gauge needle or the end of
     an opened paperclip or a battery operated cautery (beware of
     converting a closed fx to an open fx)
   • A sterile dressing should be applied

# Forefoot Problems

## 15.3 HALLUX VALGUS

Med Sci Sports Exerc 1999;37:S44; Phys Sportsmed 1998;26(5):29
**Cause:** Previous injury; congenital factors
**Epidem:** Congenital and familial factors; previous injury (i.e. first MTP
   dislocation, turf toe, rupture of the joint capsule); overpronation
**Pathophys:** Lateral deviation of the proximal phalanx on the first
   metatarsal; the medial aspect of the head of the first metatarsal
   enlarges and the overlying bursa becomes inflamed and thickened
   (bunion)
**Sx:** Pain; deformity

**Si:** Deformity of the first MTP joint; may be tender to palpation

**Crs:** Valgus deformity may progress

**Cmplc:** Degenerative changes in the MTP joint and hallux limitus or rigidus may develop (see 15.5)

**Xray:** Valgus deformity of first MTP joint; degenerative joint disease

**Rx:**
- Shoes with a wide toe box; padding around the metatarsal prominence
- Orthotic devices if overpronation or Morton's toe are present
- Surgery for persistent pain despite conservative management

## 15.4 TURF TOE

The Foot and Ankle in Sport. St. Louis: Mosby; 1995, 1195; Med Sci Sports Exerc 1999;37:S448

**Cause:** Hyperextension of the first MTP joint

**Epidem:** Flexible shoes and faster playing surfaces increase the incidence of this injury

**Pathophys:** Injury to the capsuloligamentous complex of the first MTP joint secondary to hyperextension of the joint

**Sx:** Pain, especially with ambulation

**Si:** Pain with passive extension of the first MTP joint; swelling and ecchymosis may be present
- Grade 1: pain in plantar and medial aspect of MTP joint, minimal swelling
- Grade 2: increased pain, swelling and ecchymosis
- Grade 3: severe pain, marked swelling and ecchymosis

**Crs:** Gradual improvement with treatment

**Cmplc:** Persistent pain; joint instability

**DiffDx:** Gout, MTP OA (see 15.5), sesamoiditis (see 15.6)

**Xray:** Usually negative; small avulsion fracture may be present

**Rx:** Rest, ice, elevation, NSAIDs
- Grade 1: shoe with stiff sole or orthoses with Morton's extension; taping
- Grade 2: same as grade 1; return to activity when sx diminish (1–2 weeks)
- Grade 3: crutches for several days; orthoses with Morton's extension; physical therapy modalities; return to activity in 3–6

weeks; if sx of persistent pain, joint instability, and swelling, surgery may be required

## 15.5 HALLUX RIGIDUS

Med Sci Sports Exerc 1999; 37:S448

**Cause:** Degenerative changes of the first MTP joint

**Epidem:** Congenital abnormalities; osteochondritis of the metatarsal head; overpronation; trauma

**Pathophys:** Painful restricted motion of the first MTP joint secondary to degenerative changes

**Sx:** Pain with walking or running

**Si:** Pain and swelling of the first MTP joint; restricted extension; pain with forced extension; palpable bony ridge along the dorsal aspect of the joint

**Crs:** Pain with activity may increase as degenerative changes progress

**Cmplc:** Tendonitis, plantar fasciitis (see 15.15), or other injury secondary to compensation for altered gait

**DiffDx:** Turf toe (see 15.4), sesamoiditis (see 15.6)

**Xray:** Bony exostoses and degenerative joint disease

**Rx:**
- Shoes with wide toe box and rigid sole
- NSAIDs
- Rocker bottom shoe
- Surgery

## 15.6 SESAMOID PROBLEMS

Med Sci Sports Exerc 1999;37:S448; Am Fam Phys 1996;54:592

**Cause:** Acute or overuse injury

**Epidem:** Repetitive stress or landing on the first MTP joint; increased incidence with pes cavus

**Pathophys:** Inflammation or fracture of one of the sesamoids; sesamoiditis: tendonitis, bursitis or chondromalacia; sesamoid stress fracture: similar to sesamoiditis, with persistent pain despite conservative management; positive bone scan; acute fracture:

usually a transverse compression fracture of the medial sesamoid caused by landing on the ball of the foot

**Sx:** Acute or insidious onset of pain; pain with toe-off

**Si:** Pain on palpation of one of the sesamoids (typically medial); swelling may be present; painful and possibly restricted extension of the great toe

**Crs:** Persistent or worsening symptoms without treatment; often requires prolonged course of treatment

**Cmplc:** Persistent pain despite treatment; nonunion of fracture

**DiffDx:** Tendonitis, 1st MTP OA (see 15.5)

**Xray:** Sesamoid view may demonstrate an acute fracture or stress fracture that has been present for several weeks; bone scan or CT is useful if plain radiographs are negative but sx are suggestive of an acute or stress fracture

**Rx:**

*Sesamoiditis:*
- Ice
- NSAIDs
- Padding to unload the first metatarsal head
- Semi-rigid orthoses

*Sesamoid Stress Fracture:*
- Short leg walking cast for 6 weeks
- Use of orthoses to unload the metatarsal head upon return to sports; acute sesamoid fracture: short leg walking cast for 6 weeks or taping toe in neutral position, with padding proximal to the sesamoids and use of a wooden soled postoperative shoe; if there is nonunion of a fracture, and/or persistent pain, surgical excision or partial excision may be necessary

## 15.7 MORTON'S NEUROMA

Med Sci Sports Exerc 1999;37:S448; Phy Sportsmed 1998;26(5):31; Am Fam Phys 1997;55:1866

**Cause:** Repetitive microtrauma

**Epidem:** Trauma occurs during toe-off phase of running or with repetitive episodes of rising on toes; most commonly between the 3rd and 4th metatarsal heads

**Pathophys:** Repetitive microtrauma of the interdigital nerve at the distal edge of the intermetatarsal ligament in the narrow intermetatarsal space causes perineural fibrosis; the nerve is stressed as the third metatarsal dorsiflexes more than the 4th metatarsal

**Sx:** Complaint of plantar or forefoot burning, cramping or pain; numbness in toes

**Si:** Tenderness with squeezing the web space (most commonly the third web space, occasionally the second); a palpable clicking may be noted when the thumb is rolled distally into the interspace from the metatarsal head level on the plantar aspect; movement of the neuroma over the intermetatarsal ligament produces a painful click (Mulder's sign)

**Cmplc:** Chronic pain and dysesthesias

**DiffDx:** Metatarsal stress fracture (see 15.11), Freiberg's infarction (see 15.8)

**Xray:** Unremarkable

**Rx:** Shoes with wide toe box; metatarsal pad in the affected web space; NSAIDs; one or two steroid injections; if symptoms persist, surgery

## 15.8 FREIBERG'S INFARCTION

Med Sci Sports Exerc 1999;37:S470; Phy Sportsmed 1999;27(1):91

**Cause:** Repetitive microtrauma; hypermobile first metatarsal

**Epidem:** Typical age at presentation is 13 years; 75% are female

**Pathophys:** Avascular necrosis of the second metatarsal epiphysis

**Sx:** Pain with activities

**Si:** Pain on palpation of head of second metatarsal (less commonly 3rd, 4th, or 5th)

**Crs:** Usually self-limited

**Cmplc:** Chronic pain, accelerated OA

**DiffDx:** Metatarsal stress fx (see 15.11), metatarsalgia, Morton's neuroma (see 15.7)

**Xray:** Osteosclerosis progressing to osteolysis of the metatarsal head

**Rx:** Orthoses; short leg cast for severe pain; physical therapy to restore joint motion; rarely needs surgery

## 15.9 PHALANGEAL FRACTURE

Primary Care Sports Medicine. Dubuque, IA: Brown & Benchmark;
    1993, p 448; Phy Sportsmed Oct 1996;24:58
**Cause:** Trauma; jamming or stubbing
**Epidem:** Uncommon in great toe
**Pathophys:** Bone is unable to withstand the energy generated by trauma
**Sx:** History of trauma; pain; swelling
**Si:** Pain, swelling, deformity, ecchymosis
**Crs:** Fracture healing
**Cmplc:** Malunion or nonunion; open fracture
**Xray:** Confirm fracture
**Rx:** Uncomplicated fracture: buddy taping with padding between toes;
    shoe with stiff sole and wide toe box; refer: large intra-articular
    fracture, severely displaced fracture, open fracture

## 15.10 METATARSAL FRACTURE

Med Sci Sports Exerc 1999;37:S448
**Cause:** Due to direct trauma or inversion/eversion of the forefoot
**Pathophys:** Bone is unable to withstand the energy generated either
    directly or indirectly
**Sx:** History of trauma; pain; swelling
**Si:** Localized tenderness, swelling, crepitus, ecchymosis
**Crs:** Fracture healing
**Cmplc:** Malunion or nonunion; open fracture
**DiffDx:** Lisfranc joint injury (see 15.14), tendonitis, midfoot OA
**Xray:** Direct trauma produces transverse or short oblique fracture;
    indirect trauma produces spiral fracture
**Rx:** Comfort and protection: cast, post-op shoe, strapping; multiple
    fractures: short leg walking cast; refer: first metatarsal fractures
    (significant weight-bearing role), displaced fractures (bone ends
    have shifted relative to one another), fractures at base of
    metatarsals (beware of Lisfranc fracture dislocation)

**FOOT PROBLEMS**

## 15.11 METATARSAL STRESS FRACTURE

Med Sci Sports Exerc 1999;37:S448; Phy Sportsmed 1998;26(5):31
**Cause:** Recurrent microtrauma
**Epidem:** Common in running and jumping sports
**Pathophys:** Secondary repetitive activities (running, aerobics, etc.); often associated with increased training; other contributing factors include inadequate shoes, training surface, biomechanical abnormalities, and osteopenia; most commonly occur in second metatarsal, followed by the third metatarsal; the first metatarsal is the most mobile and the second is the most stable, making the latter susceptible to stress
**Sx:** Aching or pain in the forefoot with activity, often associated with a sudden increase in training
**Si:** Localized tenderness on palpation of metatarsal
**Cmplc:** Complete fracture
**DiffDx:** Tendonitis
**Xray:** Initially normal; after 2 weeks: periosteal reaction, callus formation, cortical thickening, cortical interruption may be seen
**Rx:** Minimal discomfort: limitation of weight-bearing activity; post-op shoe or strapping; nonweight-bearing cross training (swimming, cycling, pool running, etc.); determine and correct cause of injury; gradual return to activities; severe pain: short leg walking cast for 4–6 weeks

## 15.12 FIFTH METATARSAL FRACTURE

The Foot and Ankle in Sport. St. Louis: Mosby; 1995, p 81; Phy Sportsmed 1998;26(2):47; Am Fam Phys 1996;54:592
**1. Acute fracture without evidence of pre-existing injury** (history of pain or changes on radiographs)
**Cause:** Direct trauma or inversion injury
**Epidem:** Fairly common injury
**Pathophys:** Inversion injury of forefoot: spiral fracture of shaft; inversion injury of ankle: avulsion fracture of base of metatarsal
**Sx:** History of trauma; pain
**Si:** Localized tenderness, swelling, ecchymosis, crepitus

**Crs:** Healing fracture

**Cmplc:** Malunion or nonunion; open fracture

**Xray:** Clean fracture line; avulsion fracture is at right angle to shaft of metatarsal (apophysis seen in 8–12 yr olds is longitudinally oriented)

**Rx:**
- Fracture of shaft: short leg walking cast for 4–6 weeks; displaced fracture should be referred
- Avulsion fracture: strapping and post-op shoe

## 2. Fracture with evidence of pre-existing injury (Jones fracture)

**Cause:** Repetitive microtrauma

**Epidem:** Often complain of pain prior to acute injury

**Pathophys:** Repetitive microtrauma (see metatarsal stress fracture); Jones fracture is a stress fracture of the proximal diaphysis of the fifth metatarsal

**Sx:** Pain in the proximal fifth metatarsal with weight-bearing activities; may complain of a pop or sudden onset of severe pain

**Si:** Localized tenderness on palpation

**Cmplc:** High incidence of delayed union or nonunion

**Xray:** Transverse proximal diaphyseal fracture; look for pre-existing stress reaction: radioluscent fracture line; periosteal reaction; callus formation with sclerosis

**Rx:**
- Discuss all cases with orthopedic surgeon
- Nonweight-bearing cast for 4–6 weeks, followed by 4+ weeks in weight-bearing cast
- May require surgical fixation

# Midfoot Problems

## 15.13 TARSAL STRESS FRACTURE

Phy Sportsmed 1998;26:31; 1999;27:57

**Cause:** Repetitive microtrauma

**Epidem:** Seen in distance runners and jumpers

**Pathophys:** Repetitive microtrauma (see metatarsal stress fracture)

**Sx:** Vague pain in dorsal, medial aspect of mid foot aggravated by activity

**Si:** Tenderness on palpation of navicular, usually without swelling

**Cmplc:** High incidence of delayed union and nonunion

**DiffDx:** Tendonitis, OA

**Xray:** Often normal; may see sclerotic line in navicular; bone scan will be positive; tomograms or CT will demonstrate vertical fracture

**Rx:**

- Poor blood supply to navicular and high frequency of delayed union and nonunion make this a difficult fracture to treat
- Discuss all cases with orthopedic surgeon
- Displaced fractures should be referred
- Nonweight-bearing cast for 6–8 weeks; resume full activity in 3–6 months

## 15.14 LISFRANC FRACTURE AND DISLOCATION

The Foot and Ankle in Sport. St. Louis: Mosby; 1995, p 95; Am Fam Phys 1998;58:118; Am J Sport Med 1994;22:687

**Cause:** Direct or indirect trauma

**Epidem:** Uncommon injury in sports

**Pathophys:** The Lisfranc joint is the tarsal–metatarsal joints; includes articulation of bases of five metatarsals with three cuneiforms and cuboid; second metatarsal is key stabilizer of this joint; even minor subluxation of this joint can destabilize the entire forefoot; direct trauma: foot run over by a vehicle, heavy weight dropped on foot; indirect trauma: hyperplantar flexion of forefoot with dorsal displacement of proximal ends of metatarsals, fall on pointed toes, fall backward while forefoot is trapped, sudden high velocity longitudinal compression

**Sx:** Pain often seems exaggerated; unable to bear weight.

**Si:** Pain and swelling of dorsum of foot; soft tissue damage with direct trauma; neurovascular exam very important due to potential compartment syndrome in foot

**Cmplc:** Permanent pain and disability

**DiffDx:** Tarsal or metatarsal fx (see 15.10, 15.13), midfoot OA

**Xray:** Often, small avulsion fracture is seen at base of first or second metatarsal; spontaneous reduction is not uncommon; normal AP:

first metatarsal aligns with first cuneiform laterally and medially, medial border of second metatarsal aligns with medial border of second cuneiform; Oblique: lateral border of third metatarsal aligns with lateral border of third cuneiform and medial border of fourth metatarsal aligns with medial border of cuboid; Lat: look for dorsal displacement of base of second metatarsal

**Rx:**

- Recognition of this injury is essential
- It is easy to miss, refer to orthopedics due to high incidence of complications

# Hindfoot Problems

## 15.15 PLANTAR FASCIITIS

Phy Sportsmed 1998;26(5):31; J Am Acada Orthop Surg 1997;5:109

**Cause:** Cavus foot, hyperpronation, excessive training, tight Achilles (heel cord)

**Epidem:** Most common cause of heel pain

**Pathophys:** Traction periostitis at origin of plantar fascia at medial tuberosity of anterior calcaneus with subsequent degeneration and tears

**Sx:** Insidious onset of heel pain; "first step pain" or pain with first few steps in morning or after long rest and pain after prolonged activity

**Si:** Point tenderness at medial tubercle of calcaneus; may also be tender along the longitudinal arch

**Crs:** Tends to get worse over time

**Cmplc:** Rupture of plantar fascia

**DiffDx:** Calcaneal stress fracture (see 15.16), neuroma (lateral plantar nerve), tarsal tunnel syndrome (see 15.18)

**Xray:** Calcaneal plantar enthesiophyte may be seen

**Rx:**

*Initial:*

- NSAIDs
- Heel cord stretching

- Cross-friction massage (massage against the grain)
- Ice
- Physical therapy modalities
- Arch supports, heel cups, arch taping
- Counterforce bracing
- No barefoot walking
- Limit weight-bearing activities: no running or jumping while symptomatic
- Cross train in pool or on bicycle

*If symptoms persist:*
- Night splints (Am Fam Phy 1995;52:1891)
- Possible cortisone injections (see 2.10) (Phy Sportsmed 1999;27(9):101)
- Short leg walking cast for resistant cases
- Occasionally, surgery is needed for persistent symptoms

## 15.16 CALCANEAL STRESS FRACTURE

The Foot and Ankle in Sport. St. Louis: Mosby; 1995, p 81; Primary Care Sports Medicine. Dubuque, IA: Brown & Benchmark; 1993, p 448

**Cause:** Maybe related to a sudden increase in activity

**Epidem:** Usually related to sudden increase in activities

**Pathophys:** Repetitive microtrauma (see metatarsal stress fracture)

**Sx:** Insidious onset of heel pain

**Si:** Pain in posterior heel, especially with medial–lateral compression

**Crs:** Progressive pain

**Cmplc:** Complete fracture is not common

**DiffDx:** Plantar fasciitis (see 15.15), neuroma, tarsal tunnel syndrome (see 15.18)

**Xray:** Normal in the first 2 weeks; afterwards may demonstrate a trabecular linear density; bone scan will be positive in 48 hrs

**Rx:** Crutches or cast until asymptomatic, then padding (ice, heel cups); nonweight-bearing cross training; gradual return to activities

# 15.17 RETROCALCANEAL BURSITIS

Phy Sportsmed 1999;27(1):57

**Cause:** Rapid increase in activities; poorly fitting shoes

**Epidem:** May be seen in pts with gout

**Pathophys:** Inflammation of the retrocalcaneal bursa (between posterior calcaneus and and anterior Achilles tendon) and the Achilles tendon insertion; there is often enlargement of the superior tuberosity of the os calcis

**Sx:** Insidious onset of posterior heel pain that is aggravated by increased activities and shoes with tight heel counter

**Si:** Swelling between calcaneus and distal Achilles tendon; tenderness; prominent superior tuberosity of os calcis

**Crs:** Increasing pain and swelling with persistent pressure

**Cmplc:** Achilles tendonitis or rupture

**DiffDx:** Calcaneal stress fx (see 15.16), os trigonum injury (see 15.19), Achilles tendinopathy (see 14.11), tarsal tunnel syndrome (see 15.18)

**Xray:** May demonstrate Haglund's deformity (soft tissue changes of bursitis and tendonitis plus a prominent bursal projection on the posterior calcaneus)

**Rx:**

- Appropriately fiited footware may prevent the problem
- Padding of posterior heel ("U" pad)
- Achilles tendon stretching
- NSAIDs
- Ice
- Physical therapy modalities

# 15.18 TARSAL TUNNEL SYNDROME

Phy Sportsmed 1998;26(5):31; Am Fam Phys 1997;55:2207

**Cause:** Nerve compression

**Epidem:** Uncommon; improperly fitted shoes are a major factor

**Pathophys:** Tarsal tunnel: the lacunate ligament makes up the roof and the plantar surfaces of the tarsal bones and the proximal metatarsals; the tunnel includes: posterior tibial tendon, flexor digitorum longus tendon, and posterior tibial neurovascular bundle; after the posterior tibial nerve emerges from the tunnel, it splits into three branches: medial calcaneal sensory to the heel, medial plantar motor, and sensory to the medial foot, and lateral plantar motor and sensory to the lateral foot; compression of the posterior tibial nerve as it passes through the tarsal tunnel; contributing factors include joint instability, bony impingement (osteophyte, os, etc.), space occupying lesion (ganglion cyst, venous varicosity, lipoma), and biomechanical abnormalities (overpronation); in 50% of cases, the cause is idiopathic

**Sx:** Medial posterior foot pain, accompanied by burning and tingling; pain is exacerbated by standing and activity; may complain of night pain

**Si:** Evaluate foot and ankle for swelling, presence of arches, bony prominences; percussion along the posterior tibial nerve may produce a positive Tinel's sign; there may be weakness of toe flexion and loss of two-point discrimination

**Crs:** Progressive pain

**Cmplc:** Weakness; loss of two-point discrimination

**DiffDx:** Calcaneal stress fx (see 15.16), radiculopathy (see 10.2), posterior tib tendinopathy (see 14.8)

**Lab:** EMG and NCV may be prolonged; these studies may be normal if compression is related to activity (i.e., overpronation)

**Xray:** May demonstrate osteophytes or an os

**Rx:**

- NSAIDs
- Correction of biomechanical abnormalities (arch support, medial wedge)
- Cortisone injection
- Stretching
- Possibly cast immobilization
- If symptoms persist, surgical decompression

# 15.19 OS TRIGONUM SYNDROME

Med Sci Sports Exerc 1999;37:S470

**Cause:** Accessory ossicle posterior aspect of talus

**Epidem:** Os trigonum is present in 10% of population; common problem in ballet, gymnastics, and jumping sports

**Pathophys:** Excessive plantar flexion of ankle impinges the soft tissues on the bony process (os trigonum)

**Sx:** Pain with plantar flexion

**Si:** Pain on palpation of posterior ankle that increases significantly with forced plantar flexion

**Crs:** Sxs occur with less activity

**DiffDx:** Acute fracture of os trigonum or posterior process of talus, retrocalcaneal bursitis (see 15.17)

**Xray:** Ossicle is seen posterior to talus; en pointe view is helpful

**Rx:**

- Ice
- Activity modification
- NSAIDs
- Surgery may be necessary in recalcitrant cases (usually female dancers)

# Section III

## MEDICAL PROBLEMS

# 16 Neurology

## Exercise Related Headaches

### GENERAL EPIDEMIOLOGY

- Athletes are susceptible at the same rate as the general population for headaches of all kinds (muscle tension, vascular, post-traumatic, etc.)
- In addition, there are several entities peculiar to certain athletes

### 16.1 BENIGN EXERTIONAL HEADACHE

Clin Sports Med 1992;11:339
**Cause:** Excessive strain
**Pathophys:** Due to decreased cerebral blood flow following exertion related increase in intracranial pressure via Valsalva effect
**Sx:**
- Sudden onset, severe pain in a rapid crescendo pattern with dull headache
- Usually occipital
- Pain is worsened with continued effort

**Si:** Generally nonspecific
**Crs:** Symptoms last from a few minutes to several hours
**Xray:** CT or MRI recommended to r/o organic cause; has been reported to be associated with structural lesion in up to 10% of cases
**Rx:**
- NSAIDs
- Biofeedback
- Activity modification

## 16.2 WEIGHTLIFTER'S HEADACHE

Clin Sports Med 1992;11:339

**Cause:** Excessive straining

**Pathophys:** Related to either increased intra-cranial pressure (Valsalva) or cervical ligament and tendon strain

**Sx:** Sudden onset severe and stabbing pain radiating from the base of the skull and proximal cervical spine to the parietal areas

**Si:**
- Point tender at base of skull and posterior cervical structures
- Painful ROM
- Neurologic exam normal

**Crs:** Variable

**DiffDx:** Meningitis (viral or bacterial), SAH (see 16.7), common migraine

**Xray:**
- Cervical radiographs to rule out degenerative disease or structural anomaly
- CT or MRI to rule out mass lesion, vascular lesion, or Arnold–Chiari malformation

**Lab:** Consider lumbar puncture for severe or persistent sx

**Rx:**
- Analgesic measures: NSAIDs, cryotherapy, heat packs, analgesic medications, and massage
- Physical therapy for scapulothoracic dysfunction and cervical strengthening

## 16.3 EXERTIONAL MIGRAINE (ACUTE EFFORT MIGRAINE)

Clin Sports Med 1992;11:339

**Cause:** Arise with brief, high intensity effort

**Pathophys:**
- Similar to migraine with hyperventilation leading to vasoconstriction (due to decreased $Pco_2$) followed by reflex vasodilation and headache

- Contributing factors include: dehydration, exercising in extreme heat, poor nutrition, and alcohol consumption

**Sx:**
- May have prodrome
- Severe pain, short in duration

**Si:** Negative exam

**Crs:** Intense pain, short in duration

**DiffDx:** Other intense headache (see 16.1 and 16.2); intracranial mass, hemorrhage (see 16.7), infection, migraine

**Xray:** MRI indicated in general work-up of severe headache but negative with acute effort migraine

**Rx:**
- Treat as for typical migraine; NSAIDs, sumatriptan, ergotamine, or Midrin
- Prophylactic measures include: pre-exercise warm-up, good intrasession hydration practices, good sleep hygiene, gradual physical conditioning, and improved nutrition
- Prophylactic medications may be useful; calcium channel blockers, beta-blockers, amitriptyline, or low dose ergotamine to name a few

## 16.4 JOGGER'S MIGRAINE (PROLONGED EXERTIONAL HEADACHE)

Clin Sports Med 1992;11:339

**Cause:** Arises with endurance training, generally low intensity

**Epidem:** More common with deconditioned state, dehydration, hyperthermia, and poor nutrition

**Pathophys:** Vascular headache triggered by gradual dehydration and heat accumulation

**Sx:**
- Gradual onset of throbbing type headache that is usually generalized or frontal
- Nausea, vomiting, and visual changes occur

**Si:** Exam usually negative

**Crs:** Symptoms may be prolonged in duration

**Xray:** CT or MRI to rule out vascular or structural lesion for persistent or severe sx

**Rx:**
- Usually responds to NSAIDs
- Gradual conditioning program
- Ensure proper hydration and nutrition
- Avoid alcohol and caffeine

## 16.5 CONCUSSIONS (TRAUMATIC BRAIN INJURY—TBI)

Am Fam Phys 1999;60:887

**Cause:** Direct blow to head

**Epidem:**
- Approximately 15 to 20% of high school football players sustain at least one concussion resulting in 250,000 TBI per year
- Four-fold risk of sustaining a second TBI following initial concussion
- Most common in collision sports but can occur in any sport or activity

**Pathophys:**
- Mechanics of injury include both linear and rotational acceleration/deceleration (coup/contracoup)
- These forces probably result in microscopic axonal shear-strain damage in the pons and midbrain

**Sx:**
- Acute: confusion, dizziness, memory loss (event amnesia), loss of consciousness, headache, tinnitus, nausea, vomiting, blurred vision
- Post-concussion: headache, nausea, memory loss, irritability and personality changes, difficulty sleeping, fatigue, poor school performance, and inattentiveness

**Si:**
- Mental status changes including: confusion, long- and short-term memory loss, loss of consciousness
- Poor motor coordination, poor balance, or vertigo common
- Cranial nerve evaluation may show deficits with intracranial hemorrhage

**Concussion Grading:** There are several grading systems that have been published; these differ substantially in both determination of severity and restriction in return to play; it would seem

**Table 16–1. Concussion Grading Systems**

| System | Grade 1 | Grade 2 | Grade 3 |
|---|---|---|---|
| Colorado Medical Society (CMS) | No loss of consciousness, with symptoms lasting less than 15 min | No loss of consciousness, with symptoms lasting more than 15 min | Any loss of consciousness |
| Cantu | No loss of consciousness; post-traumatic amnesia less than 30 min | Loss of consciousness less than 5 min or post-traumatic amnesia greater than 30 min | Loss of consciousness greater than 5 min or post-traumatic amnesia greater than 24 hr |

appropriate to use the more conservative (Colorado Medical Society) for collision sports where the risk of repeat injury is high, and the less restrictive (Cantu) for sports where the risk of re-injury is less (see Table 16–1)

**Xray:** Computerized tomography recommended for evaluation of athletes with loss of consciousness (severe grade 2 and all grade 3 or Glasgow Coma Scale Score <15); used to rule out intracranial hemorrhage

**Lab:** Neuropsychometric Testing: Useful in detecting or following subtle cognitive deficits

**Rx:**
- Initial management involves ABCs in the unconscious athlete
- C-spine protection until evaluated
- Complete neurologic assessment and special testing as indicated
- Primary treatment in conscious athlete is protection from re-injury and second impact syndrome through return to activity restrictions (see Table 16–2)
- Patient should be reassessed frequently after injury to ensure no change in neurologic status
- May be treated symptomatically for headaches and other complaints

**Cmplc:**
- Cognitive impairment; declining school/work performance
- Post-concussion syndrome
- Second impact syndrome (see 16.6)

**Table 16–2. Return to Play Guidelines**

| System | Grade 1 | Grade 2 | Grade 3 |
|---|---|---|---|
| Colorado Medical Society (CMS) | 1st Injury: return to play when asymptomatic for 20 min | 1st Injury: return to play when asymptomatic for 1 week | 1st Injury: transport to hospital; return to play 1 month after injury if asymptomatic for 2 weeks |
| | 2nd Injury: return to play when asymptomatic for 1 week | 2nd Injury: return to play after asymptomatic for 1 month | 2nd Injury: terminate season; discourage return |
| | 3rd Injury: terminate; may return in 3 months | 3rd Injury: terminate season; may return next season | — |
| Cantu | 1st Injury: may return to play if asymptomatic | 1st Injury: return after asymptomatic for 1 week | 1st Injury: wait at least 1 month; may return then if asymptomatic for 1 week |
| | 2nd Injury: may return in 2 weeks if asymptomatic at that time for 1 week | 2nd Injury: wait at least 1 month; may return then if asymptomatic for 1 week; consider terminating season | 2nd Injury: terminate season; may return next year if asymptomatic |
| | 3rd Injury: terminate season; may return next year if asymptomatic | 3rd Injury: terminate season; may return next year if asymptomatic | — |

Post-concussion Syndrome:
- Common constellation of symptoms in the post-injury period lasting from hours to weeks; include headache, exertional headache, memory and cognition impairment, personality changes (irritability), fatigue, and dizziness
- Persistent symptoms (>30 days) warrant CT or MR imaging; return to activity should be restricted until an appropriate period after all post-concussive symptoms have resolved (see Table 16–2)

## 16.6 SECOND IMPACT SYNDROME

Clin Sports Med 1998;17:37

**Cause:**
- A catastrophic brain injury resulting from repetitive concussive injury in the immediate post-concussive period
- Results in rapid collapse and death

**Epidem:** Most commonly reported in boxing and hockey

**Pathophys:**
- Related to loss of autoregulation of intracranial blood flow leading to dramatic increase in intracranial pressure and herniation
- Typical patient is involved in a second blow to the head after sustaining a mild concussion

**Sx:** Following repetitive blows to the head the patient collapses into a coma that is refractory to medical or surgical intervention

**Si:** Coma

**Crs:** Typically dies of brainstem herniation resulting from massive edema

**Xray:** MRI or CT demonstrate massive cerebral edema and brainstem herniation

**Rx:**
- In reported cases, acute intervention not effective
- Only effective treatment is prevention
- "Sideline" physician must be diligent in identifying athletes with even minor head injuries and restrict participation as appropriate

## 16.7 INTRACRANIAL HEMORRHAGE

Br J Sports Med 1996;30:289

SUBARACHNOID

**Cause:** May be due to direct trauma or may arise atraumatically from vascular anomaly

**Sx:**
- Presentation dependent upon size of bleed
- Large bleed leads to rapid loss of consciousness and death, small bleed may present as gradually worsening and persistent headache

- Associated symptoms may include: visual changes, photophobia, nausea, vomiting, nuchal rigidity, aphasia, dizziness, and cognitive changes

**Xray:** CT scan, MRI, and/or angiography define lesion and source

**Lab:** Lumbar puncture can identify blood or xanthochromia

**Rx:** These patients should be evaluated by a neurosurgeon

### EPIDURAL

**Cause:** Arise from direct blow to head, often associated with skull fracture

**Sx:**
- Initial headache, nausea, vomiting, and disequilibrium following head trauma
- Loss of consciousness follows

**Crs:** Death occurs due to intracranial pressure causing herniation

**Xray:** CT or MRI confirms diagnosis

**Rx:** Immediate neurosurgical consultation required

### SUBDURAL

- Most common cause of death from head injury in an athlete
- Usually associated with immediate and persistent loss of consciousness
- Requires immediate neurosurgical consultation

# Upper Extremity Peripheral Neuropathies: Median Nerve

## 16.8 CARPAL TUNNEL SYNDROME

Neurol Clin 1999;17:407

**Cause:** Compression of the median nerve as it traverses the carpal tunnel formed by the radius, ulna, interosseous membrane, and the median retinaculum

**Epidem:** Most common compressive neuropathy of the upper extremity

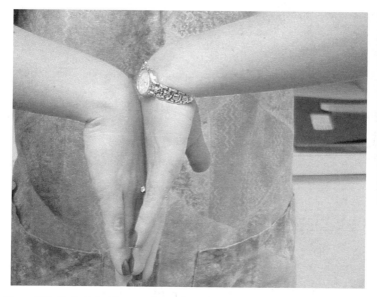

**Figure 16.1.** Phalen's test for carpal tunnel syndrome

**Pathophys:** Inflammation of the flexor tendons results in swelling and increased pressure within the closed space of the carpal tunnel

**Sx:**

- Numbness involving mid and distal palmar hand, thumb, and index, ring, and radial half of the ring finger
- Pain in the wrist and hand is also common
- Symptoms may be worse at night and frequently awaken the patient
- Frequently complain of weakness or clumsiness in affected hand

**Si:**

- Sensory changes in the distribution of the median nerve; thenar atrophy and motor weakness common
- Tinel's sign: percussion at the ulnar side of the palmaris longus tendon at the distal flexion crease increases numbness or tingling
- Phalen's test (Fig. 16.1): holding the wrist in a maximally flexed position produces numbness

**Lab:** Electromyography and nerve conduction testing are useful in confirming presence of compressive medial neuropathy and determining severity and chronicity of syndrome

**Rx:**
- Initial treatment includes bracing, oral anti-inflammatories, activity modification
- Corticosteroid injection: medication is injected beneath the flexor retinaculum at the distal flexion crease on the radial side of the palmaris longus (see 2.5)
- Surgical release of the flexor retinaculum is often required but does not exclude the possibility of symptom recurrence

## 16.9 PRONATOR SYNDROME

Neurol Clin 1999;17:407

**Cause:** Proximal compressive neuropathy of the medial nerve occurring at the proximal flexor aspect of the forearm

**Epidem:** Most common in throwing sports, weight lifters

**Pathophys:** Compression occurs at the ligament of Struthers, pronator teres, lacertus fibrosus, or flexor digitorum sublimis

**Sx:**
- Complain of numbness in thumb and index, middle, and radial ring finger with activity
- Associated with forearm flexor compartment pain
- Usually affects dominant arm

**Si:**
- Location of compression can be localized by exam
- Increased symptoms with resisted elbow flexion (between 120–135 degrees) suggests entrapment at ligament of Struthers
- Symptoms with flexion of the middle finger suggest entrapment at the sublimis arch
- Tinel's sign will localize to the level of the lesion
- Phalen's test will be negative

**Lab:** Electromyography and nerve conduction testing are useful in confirming presence of compressive medial neuropathy and determining severity and chronicity of syndrome

Rx:
- Relative rest, wrist splinting, oral anti-inflammatory medications (consider pulse corticosteroid such as prednisone 60 mg per day for 6 days)
- Surgical exploration for refractory cases

## 16.10 ULNAR NERVE

Neurol Clin 1999;17:463; Neurol Clin 1999;17:447

**Cause:** Symptoms arise from compression or stretch of nerve usually at elbow (ulnar notch) or hand (Guyon's canal)

**Epidem:** Most common in cyclists, throwers, racquet sports

**Pathophys:** At the elbow, traverses medial epicondyle beneath fascia of the flexor carpi ulnaris; ulnar neuropathy at the elbow arises from direct trauma, subluxation over the epicondyle, or due to chronic inflammatory changes of the flexor carpi ulnaris; in the wrist and hand, passes between the pisiform and hook of the hamate (Guyon's canal); in the wrist, the symptoms arise from a mass lesion (ganglion); direct trauma, or mechanical factors related to wrist position (cyclist's palsy)

Sx:
- Entrapment at the elbow presents with elbow pain radiating to wrist and 4th and 5th fingers
- Paresthesias generally involve the ulnar hand and 4th and 5th fingers and are made worse with percussion in the ulnar notch or with maximal elbow flexion
- Entrapment at Guyon's canal will involve distal paresthesias without motor weakness of the flexors (interosseous muscle may still be affected)

**Si:** Motor weakness may arise with chronic compression effecting flexor carpi ulnaris, 4th and 5th finger flexors and the interosseous muscles

**Xray:** Radiographs (AP, lat, carpal tunnel view): evaluate for fractures of the hamate or pisiform

**Lab:** Electromyography and nerve conduction testing will usually localize the site of entrapment

**Rx:**

*At the Elbow:*
- Relative rest, anti-inflammatories, physical modalities
- Elbow splint
- Surgical decompression or transposition

*At the Wrist (Cyclist's Palsy):*
- Relative rest, anti-inflammatories for acute symptoms
- Padded palm gloves, alteration of wrist position with activity
- Surgical exploration if symptoms persist

## 16.11 RADIAL NERVE: RADIAL TUNNEL SYNDROME

J Hand Surg (Br) 1998;23:617

**Cause:** Entrapment of the posterior interosseous branch of the radial nerve as it passes beneath the fibrous arcade of the supinator; frequently implicated in cases of recalcitrant tennis elbow

**Epidem:** Common in racquet sports, golf (lead arm)

**Sx:**
- Symptoms initially mimic tennis elbow with pain at the lateral elbow
- This extends into the extensor forearm and may radiate distally
- Pain is worse with gripping or wrist extension

**Si:**
- Tenderness at the radial tunnel (4–6 cm distal to the lateral epicondyle)
- Pain with resisted supination of the wrist
- Pain with resisted extension of the middle finger (localized to the radial tunnel)

**Lab:** Electromyography is useful for confirmation

**Rx:**
- Initial treatment should include relative rest, wrist splinting, and anti-inflammatory medications
- Surgical decompression considered with EMG confirmation and refractory symptoms

# 17 Adolescent and Pediatric Problems

## 17.1 SPONDYLOLYSIS

Phy Sportsmed 1996;24(9):57; Clin Sport Med 1993;12:517

**Cause:** Fracture of pars interarticularis of the lumbar spine

**Epidem:** Prevalence = 5% in general population, 63% among divers, 36% in weight lifters, 33% in wrestlers, 32% in gymnasts, 23% in track and field

**Pathophys:**
- Functional anatomy: the pars interarticularis is the bridge of bone between the superior and inferior facets; the pars is stressed by hyperextension activities
- These are thought to be stress fractures, but may exist congenitally

**Sx:** Back pain aggravated by extension activity (arching back in volleyball, weight lifting, running down hill, the follow through in a rowing stroke); usually not associated with radicular symptoms

**Si:** Usually without palpable back pain; may have tight hamstrings; pain with single leg hyperextension; stork test: patient standing with examiner behind, pt stands on one leg and the examiner assists as the pt hyperextends over the stance leg, positive is unilateral exacerbation of pain on the affected side, generally like to reproduce the pt's sx; no bony tenderness

**Crs:** Progressive worsening of pain with activity

**Cmplc:** Spondylolisthesis (see 17.2)

**DiffDx:** Discitis, Scheuermann's (see 17.3), HNP (see 10.2), tumor

**Xray:**
- Plain film oblique view demonstrating lucent line in the neck of the "Scotty dog"
- Bone scan may demonstrate focal signal in the pars

- SPECT (single photon emission computed tomography) done with the bone scan is very specific for identifying pars lesion
- MRI may demonstrate signal and or fx of the pars
- CT will demonstrate completed fx only

Rx:
- Relative rest from offending activity avoiding hyperextension and high impact activity
- May cross train with low impact (bike, swim, deep water run, stairmaster) aerobics and LE wt lifting as well as flexion biased back exercises and hamstring stretching
- Rest should be for 2–6 wks
- If sx persist or return early, consider longer restriction or immobilization in a TLSO (thoracolumbar spinal orthosis) brace for 6–8 wks
- Refer to ortho or a spine specialist for refractory cases, signs of infection, or HNP

Return to Activity: Full ROM with negative stork test; return to impact activity slowly monitoring pain


## 17.2 SPONDYLOLISTHESIS

The Low Back Pain Handbook. Philadelphia: Hanley & Belfus, 1997; p 331; Pediatric and Adolescent Sports Medicine. Philadelphia: Saunders, 1994; p 164; Major Problems in Pediatrics 1986;28:52; Clin Sport Med Jul 1993;12:517

Cause: Anterior slippage of spine
Epidem:
- 50% of those with pars defects will develop slippage
- 90% @ L5 level
- Runs in families
- Slippage usually occurs between 9–13 years

Pathophys:
- Causes include bilateral spondylolysis, pars elongation from healed stress fractures, degeneration (seen in the elderly)
- Anterolisthesis involves the anterior movement of the overlying vertebral body on the affected body (i.e., L5 on S1)
- Classification

| Grade 1 | <25% anterior slippage |
| Grade 2 | 25–50% |
| Grade 3 | 50–75% |
| Grade 4 | >100% |

**Sx:** Pain below the beltline aggravated by twisting, extension, or prolonged standing

**Si:** May have a "waddling" gait; hamstring tightness, hyperlordosis, pain with extension; may have neurologic findings (rare but usually in L5 or S1 distribution); in severe cases of slippage may palpate a step-off in the spinous processes

**Crs:** Variable, but progressive pain with more advanced and progressive slips

**Cmplc:** Radiculopathy or HNP (see 10.2)

**DiffDx:** Discitis, HNP (see 10.2), compression fx

**Xray:** Lateral L-spine demonstrating anterior slip of one vertebra on the other

**Rx:**

- <10 y/o follow exam and lateral L-spine film every 6 months
- 25% slip without symptoms may be followed with full activity
- >50% slip without symptoms should avoid high risk activities involving hyperextension or high impact
- >50% slip with sx should rest and consider TLSO brace
- Referral to an orthopedic spine specialist for persistent sx >1 yr, neurologic sx, progressive slippage, or high grade asymptomatic slips desiring to participate in high risk activity

**Return to Activity:** Good hamstring flexibility; no pain with single leg hyperextension; pt and parents understand risks and will return if increasing symptoms

## 17.3 SCHEUERMANN'S KYPHOSIS

The Low Back Pain Handbook. St Louis: Mosby, 1997, p 336; Major Problems in Pediatrics 1986;28:52; Pediatric and Adolescent Sports Medicine. Saunders, 1994; p 170

**Cause:** Wedging of three or more consecutive vertebrae of at least 5° and/or kyphosis >35°

**Epidem:** 0.4–8.3% of population; most common in boys 13–17; classic Scheuermann's occurs between T7–10

**Pathophys:**
- Functional anatomy: lumbar and thoracic vertebral end plates (epiphyses) above and below each vertebral body
- Developmental collapse of this epiphysis
- Schmorl's nodes; may be anterior or central; represent herniation of nucleus pulposus through the end plate

**Sx:** Back pain with forward bend; may not be painful

**Si:** Increased thoracic kyphosis; normal neuro exam

**Crs:** Progression is variable

**Cmplc:** Chronic pain and deformity (kyphosis)

**DiffDx:** Compression fracture, postural problem (round back), discitis, tumor, osteomyelitis

**Xray:** Irregular vertebral endplates, Schmorl's nodes, anterior wedging >5° of three or more consecutive thoracic vertebrae or one or more in thoracolumbar Scheuermann's

**Rx:**
- <35° or thoracolumbar: lumbar flexion exercises; flexibility of anterior soft tissue (pects)
- >45° brace (TLSO or Milwaukee Brace) worn 16–18 hr/d; may come out for sports activity
- >60° surgical management
- Referral for all cases >35° is prudent

**Return to Activity:** Pain–free ROM; no sport activity for 1 yr after surgical fusion for more advanced cases

---

# 17.4 OSTEOCHONDRITIS DESSICANS (OCD) OF THE KNEE

Phy Sportmed 1998;26(8):31; Clin Sport Med 1997;16:157; Ped Clin No Am 1996;43:1067; Sports Medicine: The School-Age Athlete, 2nd ed. Philadelphia: Saunders, 1996; p 273

**Cause:** Cause is currently thought to be multifactorial

**Epidem:**
- Approximately 15 to 30 cases per 100,000
- Most frequently between ages 13 to 21
- Males are affected at least twice as often as females
- Bilateral in 20–30% of cases

- Juvenile and adult onset; juvenile OCD occurs in patients with open epiphyseal plate; adult OCD is seen in patients with a closed physis

**Pathophys:**

- Exact pathophysiology unknown; the five suggested theories are ischemia, genetic predisposition, abnormal ossification, trauma, and cyclical strain
- Regardless of the cause, the result is a partial or complete separation of a segment of normal hyaline cartilage
- The plane of separation varies but is most commonly just below the subchondral plate, creating an osteochondral fragment
- Typically lesions progress through four stages; intervention at any stage can arrest the process
- About 80–85% of cases occur on the medial condyle, with the majority classically located on the lateral aspect within the intercondylar notch; the lateral femoral condyle and patella are less commonly affected

**Sx:**

- Knee pain, often vague and diffuse
- Intensity of pain often related to activity level often with swelling
- If a loose body is present, patients may present with catching, locking, or giving way

**Si:** May or may not have effusion; thigh atrophy and positive meniscal tests

**Crs:**

- The prognosis varies
- In situ lesions may heal spontaneously or progress to eventually become dislodged, forming a loose body within the joint
- Skeletally immature patients frequently only require conservative management whereas skeletally mature patients or those with a loose body generally require surgical intervention

**Cmplc:** OCD in adults is more likely to progress to osteoarthritis, intra-articular loose bodies, chronic pain, and disability

**DiffDx:** Fracture, neoplasm, ligamentous injury, meniscal injury (see 12.3), retropatellar knee pain (see 12.8)

**Xray:**

- Well-delineated lesion in the subchondral bone best seen on tunnel view
- Bone scans can help with establishing a diagnosis and prognosis because a relationship exists between radionuclide uptake and healing potential

- MRI is particularly helpful in distinguishing between stage 2 and 3 lesions

Rx:
- Varies depending on stage of lesion and skeletal maturity
- Intervention at any stage may arrest process
- Stage 1 and 2 lesions activity modification, nonweight bearing and immobilization
- Stages 3 and 4 lesions should be referred for arthroscopy
- Refer all patients with loose bodies and/or skeletal maturity

## 17.5 OSTEOCHONDRITIS DESSICANS (OCD) OF THE ELBOW (PANNER'S)

Am J Orthop 1998;27:90; Phys Sportsmed 1997;25(3):85; AAOS Instr Course Lect 1999;48:393

**Cause:** Repetitive trauma through throwing or repetitive axial loading in a skeletally immature elbow

**Epidem:**
- Males greater than females
- Typically the dominant arm of adolescent baseball players (particularly pitchers) and gymnasts
- Also seen in weightlifting, racquet sports, and cheerleading
- Panner's disease (osteochondrosis of the capitellum) usually affects children under age 10, characterized by endochondral ossification typically of the entire epiphysis, may occur spontaneously

**Pathophys:**
- Throwing or repetitive axial loading causes a large tensile force on the medial side of the elbow as well as a compressive force on the lateral side (radiocapitellar articulation), leading to microfracture and eventual avascular necrosis
- Usually occurs at the lateral or central portion of the capitellum, although lesions of the trochlea, radial head, and olecranon fossa have also been reported
- The OCD lesion or fragment of articular surface containing both articular cartilage and subchondral bone may remain in situ or detach and form a loose body

**Sx:**
- Decreased athletic performance (decreased velocity and distance of throws)
- Elbow pain with activities
- Stiffness and inability to fully straighten elbow
- May progress to repeated locking episodes

**Si:**
- Tenderness to palpation capitellum
- Decreased elbow range of motion (normal is full extension or 10° hyperextension to 150° flexion, 90° supination and pronation)
- Occasional swelling and radial–humeral joint crepitus

**Crs:**
- Dependent on size and if displacement has occurred; smaller in situ lesions will typically heal with a break from the offending activity
- Continued repetitive stress will lead to progression of disease to include: decreased performance and range of motion (flexion, extension, and pronation), loose body formation, early degenerative changes

**Cmplc:** Limited function, degenerative arthritis

**DiffDx:** Musculotendinous injuries: lateral or medial epicondylitis (see 7.1 and 7.2), biceps or triceps tendonitis; true "Little League elbow": medial epicondyle stress lesion, medial epicondylar avulsion; less likely: tumor, infectious or inflammatory arthritis

**Lab:** Normal WBC, ESR

**Xray:**
- Cystic lesion or radiolucency within the humeral capitellum, may include loose body and hypertrophy of the radial head
- If plain film is unable to detect osteochondral injury and high index of suspicion, consider MRI or arthrogram

**Rx:**
- Nondisplaced lesions may heal with rest and protection (avoid throwing, vaulting, and floor exercises in gymnastics until pain has resolved and full motion has returned)
- Lesions that are loose or partially detached may be reattached by internal fixation
- Displaced lesions should be surgically excised and curettage of the base of the defect performed

# Apophysitis

## 17.6 OSGOOD–SCHLATTER DISEASE (OSD)

Phy Sportsmed 1998;26(3):29; Pediatric and Adolescent Sports
Medicine. Philadelphia: Saunders, 1994; p 320

**Cause:** Inflammation of the apophysis of the tibial tubercle

**Epidem:** Osgood–Schlatter is most common knee complaint in children
with a prevalence of 21% in athletic adolescents; presents in girls
8–13 and boys 10–15 years

**Pathophys:** Apophyses are growth centers at the insertion of major
tendons and ligaments into bone; poor flexibility and recurrent
traction of the muscle–tendon unit causes microfractures of this
growth center during the growth spurt

**Sx:** Pain at tibia tuberosity with activity

**Si:** Painful swelling of tibial tuberosity; no joint line tenderness

**Crs:** Recurrent pain with increased activity reduced by rest

**Cmplc:** Avulsion of tubercle; painful ossicle requiring surgical excision;
permanent prominence of the tubercle

**DiffDx:** Patellar tendonitis (see 12.9), tumor proximal tibia, knee OCD
(see 17.4), Sinding–Larsen–Johansson (see 17.7), patellofemoral
pain syndrome (see 12.8)

**Xray:** Lateral radiograph demonstrating fragmentation or irregular
ossification of the tibial tubercle

**Rx:**
- Relative rest from high impact activity for short period (1–4 days)
- Ice for pain control (ice massage or apply bag of frozen peas or
corn for 20 min after activity)
- Resume activity as tolerated
- Hamstring and quad stretching
- Consider Cho-Pat strap (patellar tendon counter-force brace) for
activity
- Consider immobilization or short use of crutches for severe episodes
of pain

**Return to Activity:** Limited by pain; may need repeated episodes of
decreased activity during more active seasons of the year

## 17.7 SINDING–LARSEN–JOHANSSON (SLJ)

Pediatric and Adolescent Sports Medicine. Philadelphia: Saunders, 1994;
  p 325

**Cause:** Apophysitis of the inferior pole of the patella

**Epidem:** Preteen boys (10–12 y/o)

**Pathophys:** Persistent traction at the immature inferior patellar pole
  leading to calcification and ossification

**Sx:** Activity-related anterior knee pain esp. with high impact activities
  (running and jumping)

**Si:** Pain, swelling, and tenderness at the inferior pole of the patella; may
  have hamsting tightness

**Crs:** Self-limiting

**Cmplc:** Chronic pain, patellar tendon avulsion

**DiffDx:** RPPS (see 12.8), OCD (see 17.4), Osgood–Schlatter (see 17.6);
  patellar stress fracture

**Xray:** Usually normal or may demonstrate calcification or elongation of
  the inferior pole of the patella; may demonstrate bipartite patella

**Rx:**

- Activity moderation when symptomatic
- Ice massage (15 min) or application of crushed ice in a bag (or
  frozen vegetables) for post-activity pain
- Prn use of NSAIDs in age-appropriate doses
- Consider a Cho-Pat patellar tendon counter-force brace or neoprene
  knee sleeve

**Return to Activity:** As tolerated, limited by pain

## 17.8 SEVER'S DISEASE

Pediatric and Adolescent Sports Medicine. Philadelphia: Saunders, 1994;
  p 95; Foot and ankle problems in the young athlete, Med Sci Sport
  Ex 1999;37:S470

**Cause:** Inflammation and pain in the os calcis apophysis (insertion of
  Achilles tendon)

**Epidem:** Common in 9–12 y/o range and those involved in high impact
  activities (gymnastic, soccer, running)

**Pathophys:** Apophyses are growth centers at the insertion of major tendons and ligaments into bone; poor flexibility and recurrent traction of the muscle–tendon unit causes microfractures of this growth center during the growth spurt

**Sx:** Posterior heel pain with activity

**Si:** Posterior heel pain along the sides at the insertion of the Achilles

**Crs:** Usually self-limiting with symptoms related to level of impact activity

**Cmplc:** Chronic pain; avulsion

**DiffDx:** Calcaneal stress fracture (see 15.16), plantar fasciitis (see 15.15), tarsal tunnel (see 15.18), retrocalcaneal bursitis (see 15.17)

**Xray:** Lateral calcaneal view may demonstrate irregular contour of apophysis; consider bone scan or MRI to r/o stress fx

**Rx:**
- Relative rest from high impact activity
- Ice massage or applied crushed ice in a bag or frozen vegetables in a bag for post-activity pain
- Prn use of age-appropriate dose NSAIDs or Tylenol
- Aggressive heel cord stretching: wall stretch of gastroc-soleus, hold 20 sec 5 times per session and repeat 5 times per day
- Consider Tulley heel cup for activity
- Consider physical therapy for modalities

**Return to Activity:** As tolerated; good heel cord stretch with slow return to high impact activity

## 17.9 MEDIAL ELBOW APOPHYSITIS (LITTLE LEAGUE ELBOW)

Pediatric and Adolescent Sports Medicine. Philadelphia: Saunders, 1994; p 250

**Cause:** Throwing in baseball (esp. curve balls)

**Epidem:** The term "Little League elbow" is a group of elbow diagnoses including:
- Medial epicondylar fragmentation and avulsion
- Delayed or accelerated apophyseal growth of the medial epicondyle
- OCD of the capitellum (see 17.5)
- Osteochondrosis of the radial head
- Hypertrophy of the ulnar and olecranon apophyses

May also be seen in gymnasts

**Pathophys:**
- In children, ligaments are stronger than cartilaginous growth centers
- Apophyses are growth centers at the insertion of major tendons and ligaments into bone
- Valgus stress from the throwing motion places a stretching stress on the medial elbow
- The strong ulnar collateral ligament takes origin on the medial epicondyle (epiphysis) and inserts on the ulna

**Sx:** Medial elbow pain with activity or at night, and with ADLs for more severe cases; try to quantitate throwing (innings pitched, types of pitches, changes in training or game schedule); query for prior or co-existent wrist, shoulder, or back problems

**Si:**
- Observe ROM (may have a flexion contracture in the affected elbow for chronic irritation and contracture of the anterior joint capsule): have patient elevate arms to side with elbows fully extended and compare R to L
- Observe for atrophy of muscles (flexor group) or hypertrophy of medial epicondyle
- Tenderness over the medial epicondyle
- Pain or laxity with valgus stress (see 7.6)
    Examiner stabilizes the elbow with one hand with the elbow flexed 90° and then applies a valgus (away from the midline) stress observing for laxity or pain and compare to opposite side
    Check for evidence of ulnar nerve subluxation or tenderness (Tinel's) in the ulnar groove of the medial elbow

**Crs:** Progressive if not adequately rested

**Cmplc:** Avulsion of medial epicondyle, other components of the "Little League elbow," loose body

**DiffDx:** Referred pain from neck or shoulder problems, occult fracture

**Xray:**
- Plain films may demonstrate fragmentation, breaking, or enlargement of the medial epicondyle; compare right to left to observe for change; may see a loose body
- MRI may well demonstrate inflammation of the medial epicondylar apophysis
- CT usually indicated for evaluation of loose bodies

**Rx:**
- Initial rest for 4–6 wks from throwing
- Ice massage and NSAIDs or Tylenol for pain

- Splinting for very severe cases (short duration)
- Stretching of anterior capsular contractures: through physical therapy modalities or apply heat for 10 min and then place a small weight in the hand with elbow resting on a table and stretch the anterior joint capsule
- After 6–8 wks of rest, start strengthening and a very slowly progressive throwing program or other sport activity

**Return to Activity:** Pain-free ROM; no pain with valgus stress of the elbow; no laxity; 85% strength


# 17.10 SLIPPED CAPITAL FEMORAL EPIPHYSIS (SCFE)

Phy Sportmed 96;24(1):69; Pediatric and Adolescent Sports Medicine 1994; Saunders, p 281

**Cause:** Shearing failure of the proximal femoral epiphysis

**Epidem:** M > F almost 3:1; bilateral >50%; usually 11–16 y/o; obese or tall and thin pts; 4% with a positive family history

**Pathophys:** Weakened physis during the growth spurt; participation in impact activity

**Sx:** Painful weight bearing or limp with pain isolated to anterior groin, thigh, or knee; 20–20% will identify a traumatic event

**Si:** Painful ROM with limited internal rotation (IR); may have shortening of the affected limb; positive Whitman's sign (passive flexion of the hip by the examiner causes the limb to abduct and externally rotate as the thigh moves toward the abd)

**Crs:** Progressive with either early complete slip or chronic silent slip

**Cmplc:** Avascular necrosis (AVN) of the femoral head (11.2); premature hip OA for chronic silent cases

**DiffDx:** Legg–Calvé–Perthes (see 17.11), toxic synovitis (see 17.12), tumor in the femur, adductor strain (see 11.5)

**Xray:** AP and frog-leg lateral demonstrating slippage to the epiphysis, widening of the physis (as compared to the opposite side)

**Rx:** When suspicious, place the patient nonweight bearing immediately until is or is not confirmed; immediate referral to orthopedics for pinning

**Return to Activity:** When cleared by orthopedics; limit activity until several months after internal fixation devices have been removed (usually done when there is evidence of physeal fusion)

## 17.11 LEGG–CALVÉ–PERTHES (LCP)

Phy Sportmed 96;24(1):69; Pediatric and Adolescent Sports Medicine. Philadelphia: Saunders, 1994; p 288; Major Problems Pediatr 1986;28:77

**Cause:** Interrupted blood supply to the femoral epiphysis

**Epidem:** Usually 4–8 y/o; boys 1:750 and girls 1:3700; familial tendency

**Pathophys:** Stages of disease:
- Edema of synovium and joint capsule (1–6 wks)
- Necrosis of femoral epiphysis (several months to 1 yr)
- Regeneration and resorption (1–3 yrs)—granulation tissue replacing necrotic bone and development of immature bony matrix
- Repair—new, normal bone generation

**Sx:** Painful limping child; pain from anterior groin to the knee

**Si:** Limited IR, ext, abduction; may have thigh atrophy

**Crs:** Depends on the age of onset/diagnosis and percent involvement of the femoral head; younger children with <50% involvement do the best

**Cmplc:** Accelerated OA of the hip

**DiffDx:** SCFE (see 17.10), toxic synovitis (see 17.12), femoral tumor

**Xray:**
- Radiograph: sclerotic or collapsed epiphysis
- Bone scan: identify avascularity of the femoral epiphysis (head)
- MRI: can identify early cases where radiograph may be normal

**Rx:** Refer to orthopedics; management may include close observation, bed rest, nonsurgical (abduction bracing or casting), and surgical

**Return to Activity:** Restriction of high impact activity until well into the 4th stage of the healing process; return based on recommendation of orthopedics

## 17.12 TOXIC SYNOVITIS OF THE HIP

Major Problems Pediatr 1986;28:52; Phy Sportmed 96;24(1):69; Am Fam Phys 1996;54:1587

**Cause:** Post-viral synovitis

**Epidem:** The most common cause in hip pain in children <10 y/o; avg age 5.9 yrs; M to F 2:1

**Pathophys:** Etiology unknown

**Sx:** Recent URI with c/o limp or inability to walk and low grade temp

**Si:** Temp up to 101°F; painful ROM with leg held in flexion and abduction

**Crs:** Self-limiting

**Cmplc:** LCP

**DiffDx:** Septic arthritis, JRA, early LCP (see 17.11); SCFE (see 17.10), femoral tumor

**Lab:** CBC and ESR to r/o septic arthritis (they should be normal); consider referral for arthrocentesis and joint fluid eval

**Xray:** Radiographs, MRI, bone scan all within normal limits

**Rx:** Close observation; consider referral for advanced imaging (MRI) or the orthopedics for eval and/or arthrocentesis

**Return to Activity:** Pain-free ROM and normal gait with walk and run; consider f/u eval with radiographs in 2–3 months to r/o LCP

## 17.13 SALTER–HARRIS FRACTURES

Pediatric and Adolescent Sports Medicine. Philadelphia: Saunders, 1994; p 149

**Cause:** Usually acute trauma, but may be an overuse injury

**Epidem:** 15–20% of long bone injuries involve the physis; UE to LE is 2:1; M > F is 2:1; peak incidence age 11 in girls and 12–13 in boys; distal radius is the most common ($^1/_3$ of all injuries), phalangeal #2 and distal tibia #3; physeal disruptions about the knee are only 2% but represent >50% of all growth arrest problems

**Pathophys:** Physis most susceptible to shear forces and is weaker than both bone and tendon/ligaments; other causes of injury include frostbite and osteomyelitis

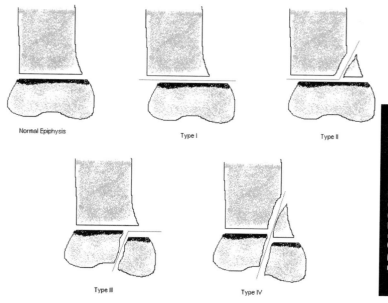

**Figure 17.1.** Salter-Harris classification of epiphyseal fractures

**Sx:** Acute injury with pain
**Si:** Isolated pain over the appropriate epiphysis
**Crs:** Depends on classification, involved joint, and diagnosis (Fig. 17.1)
- Salter–Harris I: transphyseal separation with no osseous injury
- Salter–Harris II: transphyseal separation with metaphyseal fracture (away from the joint space)
- Salter–Harris III: transphyseal injury with epiphyseal fracture (fracture toward the joint space)
- Salter–Harris IV: transphyseal injury with metaphyseal and epiphyseal fracture
- Salter–Harris V: crush of the physis (epiphyseal plate)
- Grades I–III have the best prognosis, with IV and V with worst prognosis

**Cmplc:** Growth arrest or bony bridges causing bowing of the bone
**DiffDx:** Strain or sprain, tumor

**Xray:** Plain radiograph may demonstrate widening or shift of the epiphysis with or without fracture of the epiphysis or metaphysis

**Rx:** Cast or brace immobilization; depending on the affected joint consider orthopedic referral; management depends on the comfort level and experience of the provider

**Return to Activity:** Pain-free ROM without pain over the physis or with stressing

# 18 Cardiovascular Problems

## 18.1 EXERCISE-ASSOCIATED COLLAPSE (EAC) AND SYNCOPE

Am Fam Phy 1999;60:2001
**Causes:** Exercise (see DiffDx)
**Epidem:**
- Exertional-related syncope represents only a minority (3–20%) of all syncope
- Young and healthy adults with exercise-related syncope have a greater probability of organic pathology
- In one study, 85% of EAC occurred after completion of an event; the 15% of EAC that occurred *before* completion were more likely to have an organic etiology

**Pathophys:**
- Syncope: sudden and temporary loss of consciousness associated with a loss of postural tone
- Exercise related syncope: syncopal episode occurring during or in the immediate post-exertional period; can signal sudden death and warrants thorough investigation
- Exercise-associated collapse (EAC) broadens the definition and includes athletes who are unable to stand/walk unaided due to lightheadedness, faintness, dizziness, or syncope; it specifically excludes orthopedic injuries

*Neurocardiogenic Syncope:*
- During exercise, an increase in stroke volume (SV) increases cardiac output
- Muscle contractions are crucial in maintaining venous return and end-diastolic volume (EDV)

- After exercise, lack of muscular contractions decreases EDV and SV
- This causes a reflex vagal response, leading to vasodilatation and bradycardia and, hence, hypotension and syncope

**Sx:**
- Must differentiate between true syncope *vs.* collapse from exhaustive effort
  - True neurocardiogenic syncope elicits a history of quick recovery
  - Collapse due to exhaustive effort usually presents with prolonged periods of semiconsciousness
- Determine timing of syncopal event in relation to event
  - Orthostatic hypotension *after* exercise is more benign
  - Sudden loss of consciousness *during* exercise is ominous (suggests cardiac or arrhythmic etiology)
- Other prodromal symptoms should be elucidated: palpitations (suggesting arrhythmia), chest pain (ischemia, aortic dissection), wheezing and pruritus (anaphylaxis)
- Elicit history of high risk behaviors, eating disorders, medications, and family history of sudden death

**Si:**
- Vital signs, especially orthostatic blood pressures and BP in arm and leg
- Assess for features of Marfan's syndrome (Cardio Clin 1999;17:683)
  - Tall thin stature with disproportionately long arms; arm span to height ratio >1.05
  - Unusually long lower half of body; upper-to-lower segment ratio <0.85
  - Long, double jointed fingers; elongated thumb
    - Wrist sign: thumb and little finger overlap considerably when wrapped around wrist
    - Thumb sign: apposed thumb across palm extends beyond ulnar margin
  - Curvature of the spine (scoliosis)
  - Chest wall abnormalities (pectus excavatum or pectus carinatum)
- Murmur of MVP, MR, AR/AI
- Cardiac exam with auscultation in supine, standing and squatting positions; document murmurs, clicks, gallops, and pathologic splits; systolic murmur that accentuates with standing suggests HCM

**Crs:** Benign course if found to be neurocardiogenic in origin; however, it can be a precursor to sudden cardiac death and should be investigated

**Cmplc:** Seizures, sudden cardiac death

**DiffDx:**
- Neurocardiogenic syncope (most common)
- Supraventricular tachyarrhythmias
- Hypertrophic cardiomyopathy (see 18.3)
- Myocarditis/pericarditis (see 18.5)
- Valvular heart disease (aortic stenosis, MVP) (see 18.5)
- Prolonged QT syndrome (see 18.6)
- Coronary anomalies
- Atherosclerotic coronary artery disease
- Right ventricular dysplasia
- Exertional hyponatremia
- Hyperthermia, heat stroke
- Seizure

**Lab:**
- Chemistries: electrolytes, glucose, BUN/CR, CPK (heat injuries, CAD)
- Drug screen if suspected illicit drug use
- EKG: r/o long QT, pre-excitation (WPW), LVH, RVH, ischemia
- GXT: perform *after* echo; should be sport-specific, reproduce conditions that led to syncopal event
- Other special tests: Holter/event monitor (arrhythmias), EP studies (WPW, pre-excitation), EEG (seizures)
- Tilt table testing: not useful in trained athletes secondary to high false positives

**Xray:**
- Echo: if clinically warranted, can assess left ventricular function/size (HCM), PA pressures (RV dysplasia), valvulopathies (MVP), coronary artery anomalies (left coronary ostium)

**Rx:**
- Neurocardiogenic: avoid dehydration and consider beta-blockers, disopyramide, SSRI, fludrocortisone
- Hypertrophic cardiomyopathy (see 18.3)
- Myocarditis (see 18.4)
- SVT: consider ablation

**Return to Activity:**
- If history, physical, EKG, and selected lab tests are diagnostic/ suggestive and is:
    1. Potentially life-threatening → Restriction and referral
    2. Not life-threatening → Treat or evaluate/refer as indicated
- If history, physical, EKG, and selected lab tests are unexplained, restriction from activity and perform echo/GXT:

    Referral if echo/GXT is diagnostic

    Reassurance if normal echo/GXT with reassuring, clinical features (post-exertional, nonrecurrent, normal Fhx, normal cardiac exam)

    Referral if normal/non-diagnostic echo/GXT with suggestive clinical features

---

## 18.2 HYPERTENSION

Phy Sportmed 1999;27(4):35; JNV VI, NIH No. 98–4080, Nov. 1997; JACC 1994;24:885

**Cause:**
- *Primary*: 95%; essential hypertension
- *Secondary*: 5%; coarctation of the aorta, Cushing's syndrome, hyperaldosteronism, hyperthyroidism, pheochromocytoma, renal artery stenosis, renal parenchymal disease, various drugs

**Epidem:** Occurs in 10–15% of the general adult population, and is the most common cardiovascular condition in competitive athletes. See classification in Table 18–1

**Pathophys:** Increased total peripheral resistance, which is mediated by plasma epinephrine and norepinephrine in conjunction with the effects of the renin–angiotensin system; the microvascular trauma is thought to be the cause of end-organ damage

**Sx:** Usually asymptomatic, but chest pains, dyspnea, orthopnea, poor exercise tolerance may be present; elicit family history, medication uses, tobacco, ETOH and illicit drug use

**Si:**
- Measurement of BP (JNC VI)

    Patient seated, back supported, with arm bared and supported at heart level

    Patient rests 5 min before measurement

Table 18–1. Hypertension Classification

| | Mild (Stage 1) | Moderate (Stage 2) | Severe (Stage 3) | Very Severe (Stage 4) |
|---|---|---|---|---|
| Children 6–9 y/o | | | | |
| Systolic | 120–124 | 125–129 | 130–139 | 140 |
| Diastolic | 75–79 | 80–84 | 85–89 | 90 |
| Children 10–12 y/o | | | | |
| Systolic | 125–129 | 130–134 | 135–144 | 145 |
| Diastolic | 80–84 | 85–89 | 90–94 | 95 |
| Adolescents 13–15 y/o | | | | |
| Systolic | 135–139 | 140–149 | 150–159 | 160 |
| Diastolic | 85–89 | 90–94 | 95–99 | 100 |
| Adolescents 16–18 y/o | | | | |
| Systolic | 140–149 | 150–159 | 160–179 | 180 |
| Diastolic | 90–94 | 95–99 | 100–109 | 110 |
| Adults >18 y/o | | | | |
| Systolic | 140–159 | 160–179 | 180–209 | 210 |
| Diastolic | 90–99 | 100–109 | 110–119 | 120 |

JACC 1994;24:886

No tobacco or caffeine within 30 min of measurement
Bladder of cuff encircles at least 80% of patient's arm
Two or more readings separated by 2 min and averaged
- Signs of end-organ damage or secondary causes: hypertensive retinopathy, thyromegaly, arterial bruits (esp. renal), peripheral pulses, S4 gallop

**Crs:** Chronic elevated blood pressures cause microvascular trauma; this significantly increases the risk of coronary artery disease and left ventricular hypertrophy, increasing the risk of heart failure

**Cmplc:** Renal failure, blindness, cerebral vascular disease, coronary artery disease, congestive heart failure, dilated cardiomyopathy, hypertrophic cardiomyopathy, and aneurysms

**Lab:**
- All HTN patients: CBC, lipid profile, serum electrolytes, glucose, BUN/CR; urinalysis to r/o proteinuria; EKG to r/o LVH
- Exercise stress test (GXT): may be appropriate for HTN pts age >35 with coronary risk factors

**Xray:** Echocardiogram to assess for LVH

CARDIOVASCULAR PROBLEMS

**Rx:**

- Lifestyle modifications (JNC VI)

  Weight loss if overweight

  Limit ETOH intake—no more than 1 oz per day (2 12-oz beers, 2 glasses of wine, or 2 mixed drinks)

  Increase aerobic physical activity (30–45 min most days of the week)

  Limit dietary sodium <2.3 gm of Na or 6 gm of NaCl per day

  Maintain adequate potassium intake (90 mmol/day)

  Maintain adequate intake of dietary calcium and potassium

  Stop smoking and reduce intake of dietary saturated fat and cholesterol

- Effects of exercise

  Theoretical risks of CVA with strenuous static activity due to immediate pressor effect

  However, pure static or combined static/dynamic activity may produce long-term antihypertensive effect

- Pharmacologic: when lifestyle modification fails to control blood pressure, pharmacologic therapy is indicated; there are multiple classes of antihypertensives. The sports medicine physician must remain conscious of the limitations set forth by the different governing bodies of athletics.

  Diuretics: best for the elderly and African-Americans who have difficulty controlling their blood pressure and patients with congestive heart failure; diuretics are not a good choice for endurance athletes due to side effect profile; banned by IOC and NCAA

  Beta-blockers: not recommended for endurance athletes due to decreased aerobic activity; the cardio-selective beta-blockers (atenolol, metoprolol) are the drugs of choice in the non-endurance athlete and those with coronary artery disease; banned by IOC and NCAA

  Central alpha-receptor agonist (clonidine, methyldopa): no known negative side effects in exercise; the side effects of fatigue, drowsiness, dry mouth, and post-exercise hypotension are not well tolerated by athletes

  Alpha-1 receptor blockers (prazosin, terazosin): decrease peripheral vascular resistance; best choice for the active patient with benign prostatic hypertrophy

Angiotensin converting enzyme (ACE) inhibitors: good choice for most active patients, renal protective for those patients with diabetes, most frequent side effect is dry cough; use with caution in women because of the teratogenic potential in a developing fetus

Angiotensin-II receptor blockers (losartan, valsartan): no definitive data in athletes but felt to be similar to ACE inhibitors

Calcium channel blockers: dihydropyridines are good choices for athletes, especially those with asthma; verapamil and diltiazem should be avoided secondary to their negative inotropic and chronotropic effects on the heart

Direct vasodilators (hydralazine, minoxidil): cause a direct vasodilatation thereby lowering blood pressures, this in turn causes a reflex tachycardia that may not be tolerated by some athletes

**Return to Activity:**

*Mild to Moderate (Stage 1 and 2):*
- Should not limit the eligibility in the absence of target organ damage or concomitant heart disease
- Moderate dynamic and static exercise may have a long-term antihypertensive effect

*Severe Hypertension (Stage 3 and 4):*
- Should be restricted, particularly from high static sports (see classification of sports in Table 18–2: classes IIIA to IIIC) until HTN controlled and in the absence of target organ damage
- Although inherently logical, little data exists showing exercise increases the risk for sudden death or progression of hypertensive disease

# 18.3 HYPERTROPHIC CARDIOMYOPATHY (HCM)

JACC 1994;24:880; NEJM 1997;336:775; NEJM 2000;(24):1778
**Cause:** Autosomal dominant disorder mapped to chromosome 14q
**Epidem:**
- Most common cause of sudden cardiac death in athletes less than 35 years of age
- Found in 0.1–0.2% of the general population

## Table 18–2. Classification of Sports

|  | A. Low Dynamic | B. Moderate Dynamic | C. High Dynamic |
|---|---|---|---|
| I. Low static | Billiards, bowling, cricket, curling, golf, riflery | Baseball, softball, table tennis, tennis (doubles), volleyball | Badminton, cross-country skiing (classic technique), field hockey, orienteering, race-walking, raquetball, running (long distance), soccer, squash, tennis (singles) |
| II. Moderate static | Archery, auto racing, diving, equestrian, motorcycling | Fencing, field events (jumping), figure skating, football (American), rodeoing, rugby, running (sprint), surfing, synchronized swimming | Basketball, ice hockey, cross-country skiing (skating technique), football (Australian rules), lacrosse, running (middle distance), swimming, team handball |
| III. High static | Bobsledding, field events (throwing), gymnastics, karate/judo, luge, rock climbing, sailing, waterskiing, weight-lifting, windsurfing | Body building, downhill skiing, wrestling | Boxing, canoeing, cycling, decathlon, kayaking, rowing, speed skating |

JACC 1994;24:864

**Pathophys:**
- Thickened left ventricular wall thickness, which causes an outflow tract obstruction
- Reduced compliance causes poor ventricular filling
- Large ventricular mass may outstrip coronary blood supply

**Sx:** Usually asymptomatic; dyspnea, chest pain, palpitations, syncope, lightheadedness

**Si:**
- Harsh systolic murmur that gets louder with standing or during Valsalva; heard best at the left sternal border or apex, and decrease with squatting
- Paradoxical splitting of S2
- Double or triple apical impulse
- Bifid carotid pulse (two thirds of patients)

**Crs:** NEJM 2000;342:1778
- 40% are asymptomatic and are at low risk for sudden death
- Mild hypertrophy (<19 mm): rate of sudden death <3% in 20 years
- Severe hypertrophy (>30 mm): rate of sudden death >40% in 20 years

**Cmplc:** Sudden cardiac death, syncope, ventricular arrhythmias, atrial fibrillation, and/or flutter

**DiffDx:** Coronary artery disease, "athlete's heart," valvular heart disease, pericardial abnormalities

**Lab:** ECG—LVH

**Xray:**
- CXR—recommended to rule out pulmonary disease
- Echocardiography—measurement of left ventricular wall thickness
  >15 mm: consistent with HCM
  <12 mm: normal
  13–14 mm: "grey zone"
- 24–48 hr Holter to screen for arrhythmias if diagnosis confirmed with echo

**Rx:** Depends on risk factors and if symptomatic; risk factors include: (1) symptomatic; (2) positive family history of sudden death; (3) sustained/prolonged ventricular tachycardia; (4) marked outflow tract gradient; (5) substantial hypertrophy; (6) left atrial enlargement; (7) abnormal BP response during exercise
- Asymptomatic, at low risk: defined as patients without or with mild symptoms and none of the above risk factors; consider beta-blockers, but not proven benefit in low-risk patients
- Asymptomatic, at high risk: defined as patients without or with mild symptoms and with + risk factors; consider amiodarone for prevention of sudden death, controversial; implantable cardiac defibrillator (ICD) for prevention of sudden death, consider in high risk patients, especially with >30 mm of wall thickness
- Symptomatic (CHF, Afib, syncope)
  Beta-blockers: decrease heart rate and increase passive ventricle filling and decreasing myocardial oxygen consumption
  Verapamil: decreases left ventricular outflow obstruction by improved filling
  Disopyramide: decreases gradient via negative ionotropic properties
  Amiodarone: for atrial fibrillation
  Administer diuretics and vasodilators with caution

DDD pacing reportedly reduces left ventricular outflow obstruction with improvement of symptoms; role in management of HCM is unclear

- Surgical/interventional: for patients failing medical management, or for severe obstructive outflow gradient (>50 mm)

  Left ventricular myotomy and myectomy to reduce outflow gradient

  Percutaneous septal ablation is under investigation (JAMA 1999;281:1746)

**Return to Activity:** Athletes with unequivocal diagnosis of HCM should only participate in class 1A sports

## 18.4 MYOCARDITIS

JACC 1994;24:864; Am Fam Phys 1998;57:2763

**Cause:** Most common cause is viral (50% coxsackie B) but can also be caused by bacterial infections, rheumatic fever, a variety of pharmacologic agents (lithium, doxorubicin, INH, etc.), sarcoid, radiation, and postpartum

**Epidem:** 1–7% in asymptomatic patients at autopsy

**Pathophys:** Inflammatory infiltration of the myocardium with necrosis and/or degeneration of adjacent myocytes not consistent with ischemia

**Sx:** Exercise intolerance, dyspnea, syncope, cough, and orthopnea

**Si:** Tachycardia in absence of fever, pulsus alternans, signs of CHF (S3 gallop, distended neck veins, peripheral edema)

**Crs:** May progress to dilated cardiomyopathy with chronic cardiac dysfunction

**Cmplc:** Sudden cardiac death secondary to arrhythmia, biventricular failure, pericarditis, and ventricular arrhythmias

**DiffDx:** Cardiomyopathy, acute myocardial infarction, and valvular heart disease

**Lab:** Elevated troponin T, increased CK with elevated MB fraction, increased ESR, increased WBC, viral titers, Lyme antibody titer; ECG, sinus tachycardia, non-specific ST-T wave changes

**Xray:**
- CXR: enlargement of cardiac silhouette
- Echo: dilated hypokinetic chambers, segmental wall motion abnormalities, pericardial effusion

**Rx:** Treat underlying cause, manage CHF with digoxin, diuretics, ACE inhibitors, and sodium restriction; treat complex arrhythmias

**Return to Activity:**
- Restrict all physical activity, and undergo a convalescent period of ~6 months after onset of clinical signs
- Undergo full cardiovascular evaluation before returning to activity, including assessment of ventricular function with radionucleotide angiography or echo
- Return to activity when ventricular function and cardiac dimensions return to normal and ambulatory monitoring reveals no clinically significant arrhythmias

## 18.5 MITRAL VALVE PROLAPSE (MVP)

Phys Sportmed 1996;24(7):78; JACC 1994;24:882

**Cause:** Autosomal dominant disorder of collagen organization

**Epidem:**
- 1–5% of young athletes
- 5–10% of adult athletes
- 60% women
- 4% of general population
- Increased incidence seen with autoimmune thyroid disorders, Ehlers–Danlos syndrome, Marfan's syndrome, eating disorders

**Pathophys:** Structural abnormality (leaflet thickening with elongation and myxomatous degeneration) that causes substantial protrusion of the valve into the left atrium during systole (26th Bethesda)

**Sx:** Palpitations, dizziness, and syncope, chest pain, fatigue, panic attacks

**Si:**
- Midsystolic click before a mid to late systolic murmur
  Accentuated when the patient is standing
  Diminished with squatting
- Narrow AP chest diameter

**Crs:** Surgical referral is necessary in those who develop symptomatic progressive mitral regurgitation

**Cmplc:** Bacterial endocarditis, TIA, CVA secondary to emboli, cardiac arrhythmia, mitral regurgitation, and sudden death secondary to cardiac arrhythmia; higher risk in patients with valvular deformity and/or regurgitation

**Lab:** TSH to look for thyroid abnormalities, 24-hr Holter to r/o arrhythmias, GXT to monitor exercise tolerance

**Xray:**
- Echocardiography: anterior and posterior leaflets bulging in systole is diagnostic; valvular deformity or regurgitation can risk stratify patients
- Stress ECHO for moderate–high risk patients

**Rx:**

*Low Risk:* MVP without valvular deformity or regurgitation
- Echo q5 yrs
- Education and reassurance
- Palpitations: dietary changes (avoid stimulants), beta blockers, regular exercise

*Mild Risk:* MVP with valvular deformity, but no regurgitation
- Echo q2–3 yrs
- Oral ABX prophylaxis for SBE
- Palpitations: treat as above

*Moderate Risk:* MVP with valvular deformity, and mild regurgitation
- Echo q2–3 yrs
- Oral ABX prophylaxis for SBE
- Palpitations: treat as above

*High Risk:* MVP with valvular deformity, and moderate–severe regurgitation
- Echo q1 yr
- As with moderate risk, and closely monitor function and replace valve when necessary

**Return to Activity:** Restrict to class 1A sports (see Table 18–2) in patients with MVP and one or more of the following (Bethesda Conference)
- History of syncope, documented to be arrhythmogenic in origin
- Family history of sudden death associated with MVP
- Repetitive forms of sustained and nonsustained supraventricular tachyarrhythmias or complex ventricular arrhythmias, particularly if exaggerated by exercise

- Moderate to marked mitral regurgitation
- Prior embolic event

All others *without* above criteria may engage in full competitive sports

## 18.6 LONG QT SYNDROME (LQTS)

Cardio Clin 2000;18:309; Ped Rev 1998;19:232

**Cause:** Autosomal dominant genetic disorder mapped to chromosome 11

**Epidem:** 1 per 7,000

**Pathophys:** Ion channel dysfunction affecting the cardiac potassium and sodium channels

**Sx:**
- Seizure, syncope, and sudden death provoked by exercise or stress
- Family history of seizure, SIDS, syncope, sudden death

**Si:** None

**Crs:**
- Sudden death in 30% of actively symptomatic (syncopal) patients
- Sudden death in 5% of all gene carriers

**Cmpl:** Seizures (presents in 10% of LTQS), syncope, and sudden death (presenting symptom in 30% of cases)

**Lab:**
- Chemistries, to r/o electrolyte abnormalities
- EKG

  QT prolongation; avg. 0.49 sec, range 0.41–0.60 sec

  QTc >0.46 sec approx. 93% sensitive

  QTc between 0.41–0.46 sec is non-diagnostic
- Stress test can differentiate non-diagnostic EKGs; an abnormal QT response to exercise (does not shorten) can confirm dx

**DiffDx:** Must differentiate prolonged QT from medication induced and electrolyte disturbances

**Rx:**
- 80–90% of patients respond to beta blockers; significant reduction of sudden death rates; even asymptomatic patients should be treated with beta blockers
- Implantable cardiac defibrillators (ICD) is another treatment option

**Return to Activity:** Restrict all patients with confirmed long QT syndrome from all competitive sports

# 19 Issues Unique to the Female Athlete

## 19.1 EXERCISE-ASSOCIATED AMENORRHEA (EAA)

Med Clin N Amer, 1994;78:345

**Cause:** Multifactorial including excessive training, low body weight/low body fat, emotional stress, physical stress of training; all of which lead to suppression of the HPA axis

**Epidem:**
- 2–5% of general population
- 3.4–66% of athletic women depending on chosen sport
- Most common in endurance sports (running, cross-country skiing, triathlon), performance sports (dancers, gymnasts)

**Pathophys:**
- Exercise associated amenorrhea related to suppression of GnRH from hypothalamus resulting in reduced LH, estradiol, prolactin, and cortisol release; should consider other causes (luteal phase dysfunction, polycystic ovary syndrome, anovulatory amenorrhea)
- Primary amenorrhea: failure to reach menarche by age 16
- Secondary amenorrhea: loss of regular cycle for 3–6 months after establishing a normal menstrual cycle

**Sx:**
- Irregular or absent menstrual cycle for 3–6 months
- Failure to reach menarche by age 16
- Diet and weight history usually reveals below ideal body weight, history of significant weight loss

**Si:**
- Body fat assessment: <10–15% concerning, although not definitive
- Pelvic exam: enlarged uterus, ovaries, or adnexal masses suggest other etiologies for amenorrhea
- Should conduct Pap smear and STD work-up as indicated by history

**Xray:**
- Heel ultrasound: Screening study for bone loss in long-standing amenorrhea
- DEXA scan: More sensitive and specific test for assessing degree of bone loss in osteoporosis; these tests should be considered in the initial work-up of these athletes

**Lab:**
- HCG: r/o pregnancy
- TSH: r/o hypo/hyperthyroidism
- Prolactin: evaluate for microadenoma or idiopathic prolactinemia
- FSH/LH: typically low in hypothalamic dysfunction
- Estradiol: confirmatory in unopposed estrogen states

**Crs:** Bone loss may be seen in 3–6 months, with irreversible losses in 24–36 months

**Cmplc:**
- Bone mineral loss
- Higher risk of fractures

**Rx:**
- Reduced training intensity and volume: 10% reduction has been associated with resumption of normal menses
- Increased % body fat: all EAA cases should receive nutritional counseling by nutritionist familiar with athlete care
- Estrogen replacement:
    In EAA, birth control pills are most convenient and readily available form; ensure there are no contraindications to their use
    Cyclic estrogen/progesterone may be an option
- Avoid use of Depo-Provera as birth control in at risk athletes (thin, endurance athletes, or gymnasts)

## 19.2 OSTEOPOROSIS

J Am Acad Orthop Surg 1998;6:349

**Cause:**
- In the athlete is usually due to long standing estrogen deficiency (EAA)

**Epidem:**
- Occurs in athletes in association with amenorrhea; most common in long distance runners, triathletes, gymnasts, ballet, etc.
- >1.3 million fractures per year attributable to osteoporosis in the general population

**Pathophys:**
- Estrogen responsible for stimulating normal osteoblastic cell function in replacing matrix; chronic low estrogen states lead to gradual loss of bone mass with normal ratio of mineral to osteoid matrix
- In EAA, 4% trabecular bone loss in first 12 months, 10% per year after this

**Sx:**
- None in early stages
- Symptoms of bone injury (stress fractures, acute fractures) in later stages

**Si:** None early; "dowager's hump" (thoracic kyphosis) in later stages; acute or stress fractures

**Xray:**
- Heel ultrasound: relatively inexpensive yet fairly sensitive screening test
- DEXA scan: detect early bone loss and report values relative to an age adjusted mean; currently becoming widely available; recommended to have base line tested on all amenorrheic athletes

**Lab:** Evaluation as outlined for EAA; calcium and phosphorus levels are normal

**Crs:** Bone loss does not fully recover if estrogen deficiency continues longer than 24–36 months

**Cmplc:** Increased risk of fractures

**Rx:**
- Prevention is most effective treatment; all female athletes should be queried regarding menstrual history; with delayed menarche or secondary amenorrhea, further evaluation and treatment with estrogen replacement should be undertaken

- With established osteoporosis, aggressive management recommended
- Calcium supplements: 1200 mg/day as calcium carbonate (e.g., Tums, Caltrate, Os-Cal) or calcium citrate (Citracal); vitamin D, 400–800 units/day, should be taken with calcium
- For severe osteoporosis, additional non-hormonal medical treatment may be added; examples include: alendronate (Fosamax) 5 mg po q AM, calcitonin (Miacalcin nasal spray 200 units/d, or injectable calcitonin, 50–100 units/d), or raloxifene (Evista, 60 mg po daily) a selective estrogen receptor modulator

## 19.3 EATING DISORDERS

Clin Sports Med 2000;19:199

**Epidem:**
- Affects up to 20% of adolescent and young adult females
- Most common in endurance sports (running, cross-country skiing), performance sports (ballet, gymnastics, figure skating), and weight class sports (wrestling, boxing); also common in Nordic ski jumping

**Pathophys:**
- These are psychiatric conditions that lead to significant endocrinologic disorders
- DSM-IV describes two main eating disorders that are common in the athletic population

*Anorexia nervosa:*

Characterized by:
- Refusal to maintain a minimal normal weight
- Intense fear of gaining weight
- Disturbance in the interpretation of their body image (lack of insight into their eating disorder)
- Amenorrhea (in postmenarchal females failure to menstruate for 3 consecutive months)
- Classified as restrictive type (failure to consume adequate calories) and purging type (consume adequate calories but purge after eating)

*Bulimia:*

Characterized by:
- Recurrent episodes of uncontrolled binge eating
- Recurrent inappropriate compensatory purging

- Occurring at least 2 ×/wk for 3 months
- Self-evaluation is unduly based on body size and shape
- The disturbance does not occur exclusively with episodes of anorexia nervosa
- Classified as purging type (vomiting, diuretics, laxative use) and non-purging (compensate with fasting or exercise)

**Sx:**
- A very high index of suspicion is required as the athlete will rarely present with a chief complaint of "eating disorder"
- May seek care due to fatigue or performance decrement; may have associated musculoskeletal complaints (such as stress reactions or fractures)
- Frequently is brought to physician's attention by athletic trainer, coach, parent, or teammates' concern
- Amenorrhea

**Si:**
- Below ideal body weight (IBW), typically with low percent body fat
- Dental disease due to gastric acid effects on teeth and gums (tooth discoloration, caries, gingivitis)
- Russell's sign: discoloration of one (or more) fingers due to acid effects when inducing vomiting
- Parotid or other salivary gland enlargement

**Lab:**
- Nutritional work-up including: CBC, prealbumin, electrolyte panel, LFTs, iron studies
- ECG to rule out associated cardiomyopathy
- DEXA scan for osteoporosis

**Crs:** Typically requires long-term therapy, relapses common, death does occur

**Cmplc:**
- Severe nutritional deficiency
- Death possible
- Markedly impaired athletic performance

**Rx:**
- Aggressive treatment initiated immediately upon making the diagnosis; should involve: physician, psychologist, nutritionist, coach, parents (if appropriate), and athlete
- Set target weight at IBW for height, age, and sport
- Serotoninergic specific re-uptake inhibiting (SSRI) medications are generally useful in treatment

- Amenorrhea should be evaluated and treated as outlined in section 20.1
- Restrict training until IBW is attained and must be maintained to continue training/competition
- Athlete, coach, parents, and team education is crucial for long-term success
- Psychological care is typically needed for extended period
- Should consider inpatient management if weight falls below 70–75% IBW

## 19.4 EXERCISE IN PREGNANCY

ACOG Technical Bulletin 1994;189:1; Clin Sports Med 1994;13:443
**Physiologic Changes:**
- Cardiovascular: increased blood volume, cardiac output, pulse, decreased peripheral vascular resistance
- Respiratory: minute ventilation increases 50%, 10–20% increase in basal oxygen requirements
- Metabolic requirements: increased basal metabolic rate approx. 300 Kcal/d
- Musculoskeletal: hormonal effects on joint laxity; altered center of gravity due to uterine and breast enlargement

**Scientific Basis:**
- Previous recommendations were very conservative and possibly detrimental to health of mother and fetus as a result
- Recommendations have not previously been based on scientific study
- Few scientific studies on outcome have been done
- Current recommendations based on known physiologic changes, limited studies, and case reports
- Generally felt that light to moderate exercise is safe and beneficial with certain exceptions (see below)

**Benefits of Exercise:**
- Fetal well being: decreased incidence of meconium births, cord entanglements, and abnormal fetal tracings; higher Apgar scores
- Pregnancy outcome: no increase in spontaneous abortions, congenital abnormalities, or placental abnormalities
- Pregnancy duration: slight shortening of overall length of gestation

- Labor: shortens first and second stages of labor
- Maternal well being: decreased pain and discomfort, decreased weight gain, improved fitness

**Contraindications:**
- Premature rupture of membranes
- Preterm labor
- Vaginal bleeding, placenta previa, abruptio placenta
- Fetal distress, growth retardation
- Preeclampsia
- Renal disease, heart disease
- Multiple pregnancy (> twins)

**Relative Contraindications:**
- Uncontrolled hypertension
- Moderate to severe anemia
- Poorly controlled diabetes
- Excessively high or low weight (gain)
- Smoking or excessive alcohol abuse
- Twins after the second trimester
- Previous sedentary lifestyle
- Pulmonary disease, cardiac dysrythmia, mild to moderate valvular disease

**Exercise Recommendations in Pregnancy:**
- Individualize based on previous activity, health during pregnancy, fetal well being, and previously listed contraindications
- Exercise should be light to moderate in intensity performed at least 3 ×/wk
- Avoid exercise in a supine position that will diminish cardiac output with specific reduction in uterine blood flow
- Because of diminished functional lung volume, oxygen availability will be diminished; important that the women avoid activity to a level that leads to excessive dyspnea
- Take into account changing abilities as pregnancy progresses; substantial changes in size, weight, center of gravity will increase risk of falls in many activities; avoid activities with a risk of falling or abdominal trauma

# 20 Gastrointestinal Problems

## GENERAL EPIDEMIOLOGY

N Z Med J 1994;107:328, Am J Gastroenterol 1999;94:1570
- GI symptoms most often reported include gastroesophageal (GE) reflux, abdominal pain, diarrhea, and nausea
- Incidence greater than 80% in certain groups of running athletes
- Rowers, cross-country skiers, swimmers, and cyclists report similar problems
- Runners have a higher incidence of lower GI symptoms vs. upper GI symptoms (71% vs. 36%, respectively)
- Cyclists had a fairly even split between upper and lower GI symptoms (67% vs. 64%, respectively)

## 20.1 UPPER GI SYMPTOMS

Dig Dis Sci 1990;35:956; Aust J Sci Med Sport 1996;28:93; Ann Intern Med 1990;112:429
Cause/Pathophys:
- Transient relaxation of the lower esophageal sphincter (LES) due to air swallowing, alcohol, caffeine, high fat foods, smoking, and many drugs
- Increase in acid production has been suggested; however, recent studies indicate that decreased gastric mucosal secretion, resulting from reduced splanchnic blood flow, is more likely
- Accentuated by NSAID use, emotional stress, or any factor that increases acid production

- Delayed gastric emptying, which is seen with strenuous exercise, may also contribute
- *Helicobacter pylori* infection should be considered in cases of chronic or recurrent upper GI symptoms

**Sx:**

- Common upper GI symptoms include belching, nausea, vomiting, and epigastric pain
- Usually experienced during maximal exertion
- May mimic symptoms of cardiac disease
- Symptoms are generally worse with increasing intensity or prolonged duration of exercise and are more severe with immediate postprandial exercise (within 3 hours of eating)
- Documentation of training habits, NSAID use, diet, and prior history (or family history) of gastritis, peptic ulcer disease, inflammatory bowel disease, or other GI problems important

**Si:** Generally nonspecific, may be epigastric tenderness

**Crs:** Usually effectively treated

**Lab:**

- Complete blood cell count to assess hemoglobin and hematocrit to ensure that there is no significant blood loss
- Liver function testing with transaminases, bilirubin, and amylase are relatively inexpensive and will help to exclude other causes of upper GI symptoms such as hepatitis, pancreatitis, and biliary tract disease
- Serologic testing for *H. pylori* is now available and is indicated in the runner with chronic dyspepsia

**Other Testing:**

- Care must be taken to rule out more serious causes of epigastric pain, most importantly those of a cardiac etiology; an ECG or electrocardiographic stress test should be obtained in athletes presenting with epigastric pain and associated cardiac risk factors (age over 40, smoking history, family history, hyperlipidemia, or co-morbid disease state) or if associated symptoms suggest cardiac origin (shortness of breath, diaphoresis, radiating pain)
- Endoscopy (EGD) should be performed in patients with recurrent or persistent symptoms in the face of treatment
- Ambulatory pH monitoring and LES manometry is considered with refractory symptoms following an otherwise normal evaluation

**Rx:**

- Should be approached step-wise in association with the above-discussed evaluation

- Most often, simple changes in diet, meal timing, and training habits will alleviate these symptoms; avoiding large meals 2–3 hours prior to training and high concentration (hyperosmolar) feeds while training may prevent symptoms; the use of low-fat, low-protein, liquid calorie, and electrolyte solutions is an effective means of supplying immediate pre-exercise calories while minimizing GE reflux; isotonic fluids tend to cause fewer upper GI symptoms and are the best source for calorie replacement while exercising
- Athletes may also reduce these symptoms by temporarily decreasing training or by alternating running with a lower-impact workout, such as cycling or swimming

*Medical Therapy Options:*

- Antacids (aluminum hydroxide and magnesium salts) are useful in the treatment of mild symptoms; these should be taken immediately before beginning exercise and can be repeated during the workout as needed
- $H_2$-receptor blockers (ranitidine, 150 mg twice a day; famotidine, 20 mg a day; and cimetidine, 400 mg twice a day) have been shown to be effective in decreasing upper GI symptoms in runners
- The gastric proton pump inhibitors (omeprazole, 20 mg qd; lansoprazole, 15 mg qd) are very effective, but have not been studied specifically in athletes
- Prokinetic agents, metoclopramide (Reglan) 10 mg 1 h prior to running or cisapride (Propulsid) 10 mg qid, reduce GE reflux by reducing transit time in the upper GI tract; these medications are fairly expensive and have undesired side effects in comparison to the other choices
- Discontinuation of NSAIDs or the substitution of these medications with a COX-2 selective antiinflammatory (Celebrex, 200 mg qd; Vioxx 25 mg qd) is usually prudent

## 20.2 LOWER GI SYMPTOMS

JAMA 1980;243:1743; Ann Intern Med 1984;100:843; Int J Sports Med 1989;10:s22

Epidem:
- 37–54% of runners experience bowel urgency either during or immediately following a strenuous workout

**Cause/Pathophys:**

The precise physiology of runner's diarrhea is not well understood, although a number of etiologies have been suggested:

- Rapid shifts in intestinal fluid and electrolytes with strenuous exercise results in colonic irritability and cramping
- Increased parasympathetic tone seen with moderate exercise causes increased peristalsis leading to rapid bowel transit and cramping
- In more strenuous exercise, sympathetic nervous system stimulation increases the release of gastroenteropancreatic hormones (gastrin, motilin, and endogenous opioids)
- Ischemic enteropathy and GI bleeding may also cause runner's diarrhea (see discussion as follows)
- Infectious etiologies should also be considered in acute diarrheal illnesses in runners

In severe cases, runner's diarrhea may result in significant dehydration and has been implicated in the development of rhabdomyolysis and acute tubular necrosis

**Sx:**

- Lower GI symptoms include fecal urgency, loose stools, and frank diarrhea
- These symptoms are usually precipitated with increasing training mileage or with particularly intensive workouts
- Frequently, the athlete is forced to interrupt the workout as a result of these symptoms

*History:* A careful history including:
- Symptom character and severity including the presence of diarrhea, melena, hematochezia, or hematemesis and their association with exercise, meals, or other stresses
- Any recent changes in training intensity, duration, or distance should be quantified
- NSAID use, the athlete's history of recent travel, and preexisting illness are also important etiologic factors
- A past history or family history of inflammatory bowel disease, gastritis, peptic ulcer disease, and other causes of GI bleeding

**Si:**

- Typically nonspecific
- Mild abdominal tenderness common
- Palpate to ensure no hepatomegaly
- DRE heme content determination

**Lab:**

- Stool evaluation for fecal heme content, leukocytes, ovum and parasites, and stool cultures to determine the presence of inflammatory or infectious etiologies
- A complete blood cell count should be done to evaluate for possible anemia

**Other Testing:**

- Further work-up may include endoscopy or radiography for chronic symptoms (see 20.3)

**Rx:**

- Reduction in training intensity or distance for 1–2 weeks, with a gradual return to the previous high-intensity workouts
- Exercise substitution and cross training with low impact (nonrunning) activities also help to reduce the symptoms while allowing the athlete to maintain cardiovascular fitness
- Dietary manipulations may be of some use in the prevention of lower GI symptoms; a complete liquid diet on the day prior to a long-distance competition or planned strenuous workout may decrease symptoms during the event
- Low-residue (low-fiber) diet may be helpful in some athletes
- Antidiarrhea medications should be used with caution due to potential side effects; antispasmodics such as loperimide (4 mg initially then 2 mg prn to 16 mg/day) are usually safe; anticholinergic medications (Lomotil or Motofen) should be avoided as they can affect sweating and increase risk of heat injury

# 20.3 GASTROINTESTINAL BLOOD LOSS

Phys Sportsmed 1990;18:75; Aust J Sci Med Sports 1995;27:3; Gut 1987;28:896

**Epidem:**

- Review of studies suggests that the GI bleeding may be distance or effort-related (dose-dependent)
- 20% incidence of occult blood in the stools of runners completing a marathon; with up to 6% reporting frank hematochezia
- 87% positive conversion rate on stool occult blood testing in runners following an ultradistance running event

**Cause/Pathophys:** Several possible mechanisms for gastrointestinal bleeding in runners have been suggested

- Running induced ischemic enteropathy; splanchnic blood flow is reduced by approximately 70–80% of normal with strenuous cardiovascular exercise. When low blood flow is maintained for a long period, it can lead to local tissue ischemia, necrosis, and superficial mucosal erosions resulting in intraluminal bleeding
- By a similar mechanism, reduced GI blood flow also contributes to the development of hemorrhagic gastritis, which is associated with GI blood loss in long-distance runners
- Another theory involves mechanical trauma to the bowel similar to that described in other hollow viscera such as the bladder and ureters; the repetitive jarring of the intestines results in serosal and mucosal injury
- Hemorrhagic gastritis may result from mechanical stress via traction forces of the diaphragm and gastrophrenic ligaments on the gastric fundus
- The relationship between nonsteroidal anti-inflammatory drug (NSAID) use and GI blood loss is not clear; NSAIDs have been associated with the development of gastritis and peptic ulcer disease; however, the studies on GI blood loss in the athlete have not shown any direct correlation
- Perianal disease, including hemorrhoids, fissures, and perianal chafing, is another possible cause of GI blood loss in athletes

**Sx:** Athletes report bloody diarrhea, melanic stools, or hematochezia

**Si:** Heme positive stool sampling on DRE; otherwise nonspecific

**Lab:** Initial evaluation as above for runner's diarrhea

**Xray:**

- Barium enema rarely useful
- Flexible sigmoidoscopy, colonoscopy, and esophagogastroduodenoscopy (EGD) to determine the focus of blood loss

**Rx:**

- Short-term reduction in training along with exercise substitution as discussed above
- In cases related to hemorrhagic gastritis, the use of $H_2$-antagonist agents (ranitidine, 150 mg twice a day; famotidine, 20 mg each day; or cimetidine, 400 mg twice a day) is very effective over the course of several days

- In endurance athletes who are predisposed to upper GI blood loss (ultradistance runners, or previous history of UGI blood loss), pre-race treatment with H$_2$-antagonists is effective in preventing blood loss
- Discontinuation of NSAIDs or substitution with a COX-2 selective medication (Celebrex, 200 mg qd; and Vioxx 25 mg qd) should be advised in most cases of bloody diarrhea

# 20.4 HEPATIC INJURY: ABNORMAL LIVER FUNCTION TESTS

Mayo Clin Proc 1980;55:113; Med Sci Sports Exerc 1995;27:1590; Int J Sports Med 1990;11:441

**Cause:** Results from ischemic insult due to decreased oxygen tension in the hepatic blood supply

**Epidem:** Liver enzyme elevations are most affected by long-distance running

**Pathophys:** The damage to the liver is readily reversible when exercise is stopped, with enzyme levels usually returning to normal within 1 week

**Sx:** Asymptomatic

**Si:** Usually normal PE

**Lab:**

- Increased serum glutamic-ox-aloacetic transaminase (SGOT), alanine aminotransferase (ALT), creatine kinase, aspartate aminotransferase (AST), bilirubin, alkaline phosphatase, creatinine phosphatase, and lactic dehydrogenase (LDH), have all been described in runners; although these can indicate liver injury, they may also be related to musculoskeletal trauma
- More specific indicators of hepatocellular injury, glutamate dehydrogenase (GLDH) and gamma-glutamyl-transferase (GGT) have been found to be elevated in long-distance runners
- The gradual serum reductions of albumin seen in ultradistance runners further support the possibility of hepatic injury in these athletes

**Xray:** None indicated

**Rx:** Although there is no evidence that these exercise-related enzyme elevations lead to long term sequellae, it would seem prudent to limit exercise until LFTs normalize

## 20.5 ABDOMINAL PAIN (SIDE STITCH)

Med Sci Sports Exerc 1995;27:623; Phys Sportsmed 1985;13:187

**Epidem:**
- The most common cause of abdominal pain with exercise
- Affects the athlete as they significantly increase their mileage and in untrained persons initiating an exercise program

**Cause/Pathophys:**
- The precise etiology is not known, but most likely due to diaphragmatic muscle spasm related to hypoxia
- Other possible explanations include hepatic capsule irritation, pleural irritation, abdominal adhesions, and right colonic gas pains
- These pains are often worse with postprandial exercise

**Sx:**
- Described as an aching sensation during exercise in the right upper abdominal quadrant

**Si:**
- Nonspecific with classic "stitch"
- Abdominal tenderness or constitutional symptoms may indicate more significant diagnosis (see below)

**Crs:** Generally resolves with improved conditioning

**Lab/Xray:** None indicated

**Rx:**
- The athlete may get some relief by stretching the right arm over the head or by forced expiration against pursed lips
- Stopping exercise nearly always results in immediate cessation of symptoms
- The frequency and severity of stitches usually decrease as the overall fitness of the athlete improves
- Exclude other causes of abdominal pain (omental infarction, bowel infarction, and hepatic vein thrombosis) that typically present with significant illness:

    These are very rare events and are generally accompanied by unremitting pain, severe systemic illness, collapse, and multisystem failure

    Most common after long-distance competition and require emergent surgical intervention

# 21 Infectious Disease

## 21.1 VIRAL SYNDROME

Phys Sportmed 1999;27(6):47; 1996;24(1):44; 1993;21(1):125;
   1987;15(12):61; 1987;15(10):135; The Team Physician Handbook
   2nd ed. St. Louis: Mosby, 1997; p 225

**Cause:** Enterovirus, Coxsackie virus, echo virus, parainfluenza and
   influenza virus

**Pathophys:** Change in hypothalamic set point to aid in fighting
   infection; physiologic response includes: increased sensible fluid
   loss, increased resting heart rate, increased basal metabolism,
   decreased pulmonary gas diffusion, decreased concentration,
   increased susceptibility to heat illness and injury

**Sx:** May or may not be associated with myalgia and pulmonary, upper
   respiratory, GI, or GU symptoms

**Si:** Temp >100.4°F; focal or nonfocal signs

**Crs:** Usually self-limiting

**Cmplc:** Untreated focal infection; sudden death due to myocarditis

**DiffDx:** Early focal infection (UTI, pyelonephritis, pneumonia,
   pharyngitis, sinusitis, gastroenteritis), CVD

**Lab:** If ordered, CBC demonstrating elevated lymph/mono count

**Rx:** Acetaminophen (Tylenol) 650–1000 mg qid; ibuprofen (Motrin)
   400 mg qid to 800 mg tid

**Return to Activity:** "Neck check" (Phys Sportmed 1993;21:125)
   resolution of below the neck symptoms (fever, severe cough,
   diarrhea/vomiting, myalgias); normal hydration

## 21.2 UPPER RESPIRATORY INFECTION (URI)

Phy Sportmed 1998;26(2):85

**Cause:** Enterovirus, rhinovirus, parainfluenza virus, influenza virus

**Epidem:** Seasonal prevalence Sep–Apr; onset of sx 1–2 d after exposure
with duration of 1–2 wks; person-to-person spread

**Pathophys:** Viral invasion of respiratory mucosa; may be related to
depressed secretory IgA or exercise-related mucosal drying,
irritation, and suppressed ciliary action

**Sx:** Upper respiratory congestion with nasal discharge, postnasal drip
with night cough, low grade temperature, fatigue, ± myalgias

**Si:** Low grade fever, nasal fullness, sinus tenderness, fluid behind TMs
or TM retraction, mild throat erythema, clear lungs, shotty
cervical lymph nodes

**Crs:** Self-limiting lasting 7–14 days

**Cmplc:** Sinusitis, otits media, pneumonia, asthma exacerbation, GABS

**DiffDx:** Sinusitis (see 21.4), GABS, IM (see 21.6)

**Lab:** Consider throat culture or rapid strep

**Xray:** Normal CXR or sinus series if ordered

**Rx:** Symptom directed care; relative rest, fluids, antipyretics, analgesics,
saline gargle, oral decongestants (Entex, Sudafed), topical
decongestants (Afrin, phenylephrine, Atrovent nasal drops),
antitussives (Tessalon, guaifenesen)

**Return to Activity:** Resolved constitutional symptoms; if symptoms
minor may consider to continue training (begin training at 50%
intensity and if feeling ok after 5–10 min, then may train at full
intensity); beware post-viral bronchial reactivity (may need
bronchodialator) (Phys Sportmed 1987;15(12):61)

## 21.3 OTITIS MEDIA

Clin Sport Med 1997;16:635
**Cause:** Infection/pus in middle ear
**Epidem:** Organisms include *S. pneumoniae*, *H. influenzae*, *B. catarrhalis*, etc.
**Pathophys:** Eustachian tube dysfunction from abn anatomy or irritation and soft tissue swelling from URI, irritants (smoke, allergies, etc.), or altitude and aquatic activities
**Sx:** Antecedent URI; exposure to irritants, altitude, fumes; travel history; auralgia, fever, attenuation of hearing, ± vertigo
**Si:** Red, bulging TM, absent movement with Valsalva; purulent debris may represent rupture
**Cmplc:** Perforation; serous otitis with effusion; perilymph fistula; chloesteatoma; hearing loss
**DiffDx:** Serous otitis; eustachian tube dysfunction, TMJ dysfunction
**Rx:**

*Antibiotics:*
- Amoxicillin 250–500 mg tid for 10 d
- Erythromycin 250 mg qid for 10 d
- Amoxicillin/clavulanate (Augmentin) 875 mg bid for 10 d
- Azithromycin (Zithromax) 500 mg d 1 then 250 mg qd for 4 d
- Trimethoprim/sulfamethoxazole (Septra DS) bid for 10 d
- Loracarbef (Lorabid) 200–400 mg bid for 7–10 d

*Decongestants:*
- Phenylpropanolamine (Entex LA) 75 bid or (Entex) 25 mg q4h
- Pseudoephedrine (Sudafed) 30–60 mg qid
- Oxymetazoline (Afrin) nasal

*Topical analgesics:*
- Benzocaine + antipyrine (Auralgan)

Oral analgesics; referral-persistent effusion, hearing loss, vertigo lasting more than a few days esp. if associated with hearing loss/attenuation
**Return to Activity:** Resolved fever and constitutional symptoms, no vertigo, resolved perforation if traveling to altitude or aquatic sports, normal Valsalva function for altitude and aquatic sports

## 21.4 SINUSITIS

Am Fam Phys 1998;58:1795; Post Grad Med 1997;102:253

**Cause:** See 22.3

**Epidem:** Organisms include *S. pneumoniae, H. influenzae, B. catarrhalis*, etc.

**Pathophys:** Nasal mucosal swelling from irritants (smoke/smog), URI, allergic or vasomotor rhinitis and impaired ciliary motility

**Sx:** Antecedent URI; altitude or aquatic activities; the URI that does not resolve; headache, fever, purulent nasal discharge, facial or dental pain, cough from postnasal drip or bronchospasm

**Si:** Fever, sinus tenderness (unilateral), foul nasal discharge or secretions, opaque sinus on transillumination; pain with Valsalva or forward bend

**Crs:** Variable depending on treatment and continued environmental exposures

**Cmplc:** Sepsis, osteomyelitis, meningitis, chronic pain

**DiffDx:** Sinus congestion/fullness, allergic rhinitis, dental abscess

**Lab:** Consider CBC for the more ill patient

**Xray:** Plain films demonstrating air–fluid level or mucosal wall thickening or CT

**Rx:**

- Antipyretics
- Analgesics
- Antibiotics for 14–21 days (amoxicillin, Augmentin, Septra, azithromycin, Cleocin for recurrent infections)
- Sinus drainage (topical Afrin or phenylephrine)
- Nasal steroids for 3–4 weeks (Flonase, Vancenase, Beconase)

**Return to Activity:** Resolved constitutional symptoms, no vertigo


## 21.5 PNEUMONIA

Phy Sport Med 1997;25(10):43

**Cause:** Lower respiratory tract infection

**Epidem:** Community-acquired organismas (*S. pneumoniae* and *H. influenzae*) or atypical organisms (*Mycoplasma*, viral, *Legionella*, *Chlamydia*)

**Pathophys:** May have antecedent URI

**Sx:** Fever, myalgia, fatigue and lassitude, cough that may or may not be productive

**Si:** Fever, ill appearing, rales, rhonchi, signs of consolidation

**Crs:** Variable

**Cmplc:** Sepsis, endocarditis, meningitis, empyema, hypoxia, prolonged incapacitation

**DiffDx:** Asthma, bronchitis, foreign body aspiration

**Lab:** CBC, ABG

**Xray:** Consolidation, infiltrate on CXR

**Rx:**

- Antipyretics
- Analgesics for chest pains: ibuprofen or codeine
- Antibiotics

  Erythromycin 250 mg qid for 10 d

  Amoxicillin/clavulanate (Augmentin) 875 mg bid for 10 d

  Azithromycin (Zithromax) 500 mg day 1 then 250 mg qd for 4 d

  Loracarbef (Lorabid) 200–400 mg bid for 7–10 d

**Return to Activity:**

- Resolved constitutional symptoms and fever
- Adequate energy level
- Generally 2 days rest for every day of lost training
- Begin @ 50% intensity 7 days after resolution of systemic symptoms with gradual increase in intensity over 7 days
- Proceed slowly and as tolerated

## 21.6 INFECTIOUS MONONUCLEOSIS (IM)

Am Fam Phys 1994;49:879; Phy Sportmed 1993;21(1):125; 1996;24(4):49; Clin Sport Med 1997;16:635

**Cause:** Epstein-Barr virus of the Herpes family

**Epidem:** 95% infected by age 25; 15–25 age group highest prevalence; only 50% are symptomatic; affect 25% of college-aged individuals; not highly contagious among college roommates

**Pathophys:** Infects B cells; transmitted by intimate contact

**Sx:** Fever, fatigue, sore throat, ± abdominal pain; possible exposure history to IM

**Si:** Tired appearing; purulent pharyngitis; diffuse adenopathy (esp. posterior cervical) signs of hepatosplenomegaly

**Crs:** Usually self-limiting, but may have prolonged fatigue

**Cmplc:** Loss of training time, school or work performance due to prolonged fatigue; upper airway obstruction; splenic rupture; Guillain-Barré; thrombocytopenia or hemolytic anemia

**DiffDx:** GABS, CMV, enterovirus, Coxsackie, GC, *Mycoplasma*

**Lab:** Mild leukocytosis with increased ATL count; elevated transaminases; elevated urine specific gravity or BUN if dehydrated; may have hemolytic anemia or thrombocytopenia; throat culture or rapid strep test

**Xray:** Consider US, CT, or MRI to eval splenomegaly in large athletes (hard to examine or those requesting early return to activity); spleen longitudinal length <15 cm or spleen to ipsilateral kidney ratio <1.25 (Pediatr Radiol 1998;28:98)

**Rx:**
- Symptomatic management of fever and fatigue
- No contact activity for 4–6 weeks
- Low impact aerobics as tolerated over first 2–4 weeks
- Appropriate antibiotics for strep pharyngitis (penicillin or erythromycin)
- Corticosteroids for significant tonsilar enlargement or elevated transaminases
- Referral for splenic rupture; airway compromise; hemolytic anemia or thrombocytopenia; consider referral of those placed on oral corticosteroids

**Return to Activity:** Resolved constitutional symptoms and adequate energy level; normal labs (CBC and LFTs); normal physical exam; negative imaging study, if indicated (see above)

## 21.7 DIARRHEA

Phy Sportmed 1997;25(11):80; Clin Sport Med 1997;16:635

**Cause:** Infection or drugs

**Epidem:** Viral (rotavirus, Norwalk agent, enteroviruses); bacterial (*Shigella, Salmonella, Yersinia*); protozoan (*Giardia, E. histolytica*)

**Pathophys:** Increased water content of stool

**Sx:** Fever, myalgia, diarrhea (watery/bloody); h/o travel

**Si:** Fever, signs of dehydration, ± abdominal pain

**Crs:** Usually self-limiting

**Cmplc:** Dehydration and electrolyte dysfunction; heat illness or other injury if training intensity while ill; sepsis; contagiousness

**DiffDx:** IBD, IBS, diverticulitis, diverticulosis, cancer, ischemic bowel

**Lab:** Fecal WBC, stool culture, consider CBC and chemistries if signs of dehydration or severe infection

**Xray:** Acute abdominal series (AAS) for signs of significant illness

**Rx:**

- Fluids (oral or IV)
- Antispasmodics
  Dycyclomine (Bentyl) 10–20 mg qid
  Phenobarbital/atropine/hyoscyamine (Donnatal) 1–2 tab qid
- Loperamide (Imodium) 4 mg initial followed by 2 mg prn loose stool to max 16 mg/d
- Antibiotics for positive cultures or for traveler's diarrhea if in foreign country (Cipro 500/d for 5 days)
- Avoid caffeine, NSAIDs, and high carbohydrate drinks/foods

**Return to Activity:** Guided by hydration state, risk of infecting others, and desire to return

# Skin Infections of Concern in Contact Sports

## 21.8 CELLULITIS

Phy Sportmed 1997;25(12):45

**Cause:** *Strep*, *S. aureus*

**Epidem:** Common in all contact sports (esp. wrestling, judo, karate)

**Pathophys:** Local soft tissue trauma (abrasion, arthropod/human/animal bite) causing epidermal breakdown and secondary bacterial invasion into subcutaneous tissues

**Sx:** Fever, local soft tissue pain, swelling, and possible drainage

**Si:** ? area of skin breakdown (abrasion, excoriation, tinea lesion), erythema, heat, induration, lymphangitic streaking

**Cmplc:** Sepsis, endocarditis, osteomyelitis

**DiffDx:** Venous stasis if on LE; myositis; muscle contusion/hematoma

**Lab:** Elevated WBC

**Xray:** Consider soft tissue film to look for gas in severe cases

**Rx:** Warm compress, elevation, antipyretics and analgesics; antistaphylococcal antibiotics:
- Erythromycin 250–500 mg qid
- Amoxicillin/clavulanate (Augmentin) 875 mg bid
- Dicloxacillin 250–500 mg qid
- Cephalexin (Keflex) 250–500 mg qid
- Levofloxacin 250–500 mg/d
- Ciprofloxacin 250–750 mg bid

**Return to Activity:** Dry or clinically resolved; resolved constitutional symptoms

## 21.9 HERPES

Phy Sportmed 1997;25(12):45; Clin Sport Med 1997;16:635

**Cause:** HSV-1 or -2

**Epidem:** By age 50, 90% of population HSV-1 seropositive; estimated prevalence in one wrestling season of 2.6% for high school and 7.6% for college

**Pathophys:** Primary infections for close contact with infectious athletes or from wrestling/gymnastic mats; may have recurrent outbreaks from prior infection

**Sx:** Skin erruption with antecedent burning pain; low grade fever; myalgia

**Si:** Clusters of vesicles on erythematous base that may occur anywhere (face, neck, trunk, etc.)

**Crs:** Left untreated, spontaneous resolution will occur in 7–10 days

**Cmplc:** Recurrent infection, contamination of sport equipment and spread of infection to others, secondary infection, scarring, neuralgia

**DiffDx:** Abscess, eczema, or contact dermatitis

**Lab:** Tzank prep demonstrating multinucleated giant cells; viral culture of base of vessicle

**Rx:**
- Analgesics
- Astringents (topical Domeboro compresses)
- Oral antivirals

Acyclovir (Zovirax) 400 mg tid for 5–7 d
Valacylclovir (Valtrex) 500 mg bid for 5 d
Famciclovir (Famivir) 125 mg bid for 5 d
**Return to Activity:** No new vesicles and all old vesicles dry and well crusted, resolved erythema, no secondary infection

## 21.10 TINEA (RING WORM)

Phy Sportmed 1997;25(12):45; Clin Sport Med 1997;16:635
**Cause:** Dermatophytes usually from *Trichophyton* genus
**Epidem:** Of concern in close contact sports (wrestling and martial arts)
**Pathophys:** Moisture and direct skin contact with infected mat or athletic equipment and abrasions allowing local infection
**Sx:** Pruritic slowly enlarging rash
**Si:** Discoid, red, raised patch, with some scale and/or crust
**Crs:** Self-limiting; slow growth; no long term sequelae
**Cmplc:** Secondary infection, spread of disease to others
**DiffDx:** Contact dermatitis, abrasion, psoriasis, seborrheic dermatitis
**Lab:** Exam of scrapings under KOH demonstrating branching hyphae
**Rx:**
*Topical antifungals:*
• Clotrimazole 1% (Lotrimin) bid
• Tolnaftate (Tinactin) bid
• Terbinafine (Lamisil) qd
• Econazole (Spectazole) qd or bid
• Ketoconazole (Nizoral) 2% cream qd
*Oral antifungals:* For refractory or recurrent cases:
• Ketoconazole (Nizoral) 200 mg/d for 4 wks
• Terbinafine (Lamisil) 250 mg/d qd for 2 wks
• Fluconazole 150 mg 1 ×/wk for 1–4 wks
**Return to Activity:** 24 hrs of therapy, may be covered; when lesion is flattened and scaling resolved

# 22 Other Medical Problems

## 22.1 OVERTRAINING (STALENESS)

Med Sci Sp Ex 2000;32:317; 1998;30:1140; 1998;30:1146; 1997;30:1173; Sport Med 1999;27:73; 1998;26:177; 1998;26:1; 1996;21:80; J Sport Sci 1997;15:341

**Cause:** Excessive training and competition without adequate recovery

**Epidem:** Affects 5–15% of elite athletes at any one time

**Pathophys:** Multiple hypotheses:

- *Chronic glycogen depletion*: chronic nutritional deficiency leading to chronic glycogen depletion and increased oxidation of branched chain amino acids and a change in the BCAA:fTry ratio and ultimately, central fatigue (Med Sci Sp Ex 1998;30:1146)

- *Autonomic imbalance*: increased sympathetic activity from stress and overloaded target organs and increased catabolism leading to decreased sympathetic intrinsic activity (Med Sci Sp Ex 1998;30:1140)

- *Central fatigue hypothesis*: peripheral fatigue and nutrient depletion leading to the consumption of BCAAs, with subsequent change in the BCAA:fTry ratio; with elevated CNS fTry leading to elevated CNS 5HT and central fatigue (Med Sci Sp Ex 1997;30:1173)

- *Glutamine hypothesis* (immune dysfunction): overload training leading to depressed glutamine production from muscle tissue; glutamine deficiency as well as acute exercise stress on the immune system create immunologic open window leading to repeated minor infections and systemic stress (Sport Med 1998;26:177)

- *Cytokine hypothesis*: incomplete recovery of locally damaged tissues with overload causing a local inflammatory response to become systemic with elevated pro-inflammatory cytokines IL-1β, TNF-α, and IL-6 (Med Sci Sp Ex 2000;32:317)

**Sx:** Fatigue; decreased performance; overuse injuries (musculoskeletal manifestation of overtraining); sleep disturbance; mood disorder

**Si:** Elevated resting HR (usually >10 bpm over baseline); decreased lean body mass; depressed mood on various evaluation tools; otherwise essentially normal exam

**Crs:** Depends on duration and severity of symptoms and the athlete's and coach's management

**Cmplc:** Early retirement, poor performance during key periods (Olympics, etc.), injury

**DiffDx:**
- Infectious disease: infectious mono, Lyme disease, pneumonia, CMV, other viral infection (see Chapter 21)
- Metabolic disorders: anemia, diabetes, hypo/hyper thyroid
- Substance abuse: ETOH, cocaine, marijuana, stimulants
- Mood disorder: depression, bipolar disorder, other
- Cancer: lymphoma, leukemia, other
- Other: pregnancy

**Lab:** Initial eval consider CBC, ESR, chem 20, TSH, ferritin, serum β-HCG, monospot; at F/U consider nutritional assessment or psychologic evaluation

**Rx:**
- Rest (initially for 2 weeks), if recovered then resume more balanced training
- More significant symptoms may require longer periods of rest from training and competition
- Upon return to activity, need more balanced training (periodization) with periods of relative rest and cross training to avoid monotony and overuse, with careful attention to sleep, nutrition, hydration, social support, and stretching

**Return to Activity:** Monitor overall recovery process and listen to the body's signals (mood, myalgias, sense of well being)

# 22.2 EXERTIONAL RHABDOMYOLYSIS

Arch Intern Med 1976;136:692; Mil Med 1996;161:564; 1989;154:244; Am Fam Phys 1995;52:502; Phy Sportmed 1992;20(10):95

**Cause:** Muscle breakdown from severe, exhaustive exercise

**Epidem:**
- Many reports associate with mass training or mass participation as in military training or police training of recruits
- Risk factors of high ambient temp and high humidity, poor conditioning, dehydration, compromised nutritional state, hypoxia, sickle cell disease or trait, medication use (aspirin, phenothiazines, anticholinergics), drugs (cocaine, alcohol), renal insufficiency, recent viral illness, or prior heat injury

**Pathophys:** Severe muscle breakdown with release of toxins and electrolytes leading to hypernatremia, hyperkalemia, hyperuricemia, lactic acidosis, and secondary oliguric renal failure

**Sx:** H/o exhaustive exercise session (often eccentric type); delayed onset muscle soreness with local swelling

**Si:** Significant local compartment soft tissue swelling; pain with passive motion of muscles; decreased urine output; may have signs of multiorgan failure or even collapse

**Crs:** Variable depending on extent of muscle damage and comorbid disease

**Cmplc:** Renal failure, multiorgan failure, compartment syndrome, ARDS, DIC

**DiffDx:** Delayed onset muscle soreness, exertional compartment syndrome without rhabdomyolysis

**Lab:** Elevated CPK, urine myoglobin (or positive dipstick for blood without RBC on micro); elevated LFTs, BUN, creat, sodium, potassium and lactic acidosis; secondary hypocalcemia, hyperphosphatemia, hypoalbuminemia and oliguria with subsequent DIC (thrombocytopenia, decreased fibrinogen)

**Rx:**
- Aggressive fluid resuscitation (4–10 L in first 24 hrs)
- Lasix 40–120 mg
- Mannitol (100 cc of 25% solution)
- Consider alkalization of urine
- Monitor and manage compartment syndrome with fasciotomy as required

- Monitor electrolytes and treat deficient or excess states as indicated (potassium, calcium)
- In severe cases of renal failure consider dialysis

**Return to Activity:** May take several months up to 1 year; begin with stretching and low impact aerobics then concentric exercise and slow advancement as tolerated

## 22.3 EXERCISE-INDUCED HEMATURIA

Am Fam Phys 1996;53:905; Urol Clin N Am 1998;25:661

**Cause:** Exercise

**Epidem:** 15–30% of runners; 11–100% of all athletes

**Pathophys:**
- Renal causes: jostling and shaking of the kidney, direct blow to kidney, increased glomerular permeability to RBC or vasoconstriction and hypoxic damage to nephron
- Bladder causes: repetitive impacts of the posterior vesicle wall against its base
- Prostatic and urethral causes: direct trauma esp. in cyclists

**Sx:** Usually none; may have discolored urine

**Si:** Gross or microscopic hematuria

**Crs:** Resolves with 24–72 hrs of rest

**Cmplc:** UTI, anemia

**DiffDx:** UTI/cystitis; upper tract disease; nephrolithiasis; STD; tumor; drugs/medication; dye ingestion

**Lab:** UA, C&S, serum creatinine, urine cytology

**Xray:** Consider IVP

**Rx:**
- Adequate hydration and keep urine in bladder with running
- Exercise moderation
- Refer for age >40, gross hematuria, recurrent sx, hematuria with no exercise, or low intensity and hematuria that does not clear with rest

## 22.4 EXERCISE-INDUCED ASTHMA

Phy Sportmed 1999;27:75; Clin Sport Med 1998;17:344; J of All and
  Clin Imm 1998;101;646

**Cause:**
- Vigorous physical activity
- Cold, dry air especially asthmogenic
- Tobacco smoke, sulfur dioxide, smog, molds, and pollens can
  aggravate

**Epidem:**
- Occurs in up to 90% of individuals with chronic asthma and in
  40% of those who have allergic rhinitis or atopic dermatitis
- Prevalence varies by sport; may be seen in 10–50% of competitive
  athletes

**Pathophys:** Unknown, however there are two main theories

*Water Loss Theory:* Normally, dry air is conditioned while passing
  through the nose, pharynx, and first seven generations of bronchi;
  with exercise, the ventilation rate increases and most breathing
  occurs through the mouth, bypassing conditioning; the airways
  become dry with alterations in osmolarity, pH, and temperature
  of the periciliary fluid; this results in mediator release and
  bronchoconstriction

*Heat Exchange Theory:* Increased ventilation cools the airways
  during vigorous exercise; with the cessation of exercise, the
  bronchial vasculature dilates and engorges to rewarm the
  epithelium; engorged vessels then narrow the airways and may
  leak, resulting in mediator release and bronchospasm

**Sx:**
- Cough, wheezing, excessive sputum production, dyspnea, and/or
  chest tightness following 6–8 min of strenuous exercise
- Avoidance of exercise in children
- Inability to keep up with peers
- Poorer performance than training predicts

**Si:** Office exam may be normal or wheezing in chronic asthmatic
    patients

**Crs:**
- Symptoms typically develop after 6–8 min of exercise at greater
  than 80% of maximum predicted HR

- The greatest decrease in pulmonary function is seen about 15 min after exercise begins
- Normal lung function returns 30–60 min after cessation of exercise
- In about 30% of patients, particularly children, a late phase or second decrease in lung function may occur 6–8 hs after the onset of exercise
- 40–50% of patients with exercise induced asthma may have a refractory period where exercise within 1–4 hs of initial activity does not induce symptoms

**Cmplc:**
- Untreated, it may result in respiratory distress
- Decreased physical fitness, possibly poor self-image, poor peer-group acceptance as a result of avoiding regular childhood activities

**DiffDx:** Bronchitis, pneumonia (see 21.5), croup, CHF, congenital heart disease, hyperventilation, cystic fibrosis, pulmonary embolism, GERD, anaphylactic reaction, bronchopulmonary dysplasia, foreign body aspiration, laryngeal webs, chemical irritation, lymphadenopathy, vascular rings, tumor, laryngeal dysfunction

**Lab:**
- Peak expiratory flow rate may be helpful during real-life event
- Exercise challenge in a lab is most precise method of making diagnosis:

  Resting $FEV_1$ 80–100% predicted; <80% predicted is indicative of chronic asthma

  5–8 min of high intensity exercise (75–80% of maximum predicted HR) without warm-up; spirometry is performed every 3 min following exercise and EIA is classified as mild: 15–20% drop in $FEV_1$, moderate: 20–30% drop in $FEV_1$, or severe: >30% drop in $FEV_1$

- Metacholine challenge test may be useful if exercise testing is not conclusive; it is more sensitive but less specific than exercise testing.

**Rx:**

*Nonpharmacologic:*
- Exercise conditioning
- Avoid exercise in cold, dry air
- Avoid triggers and known triggering exercises
- Cover nose and mouth with a scarf or breathing mask to warm and humidify air
- Appropriate warm-up may induce a refractory period
- Cool down following activity

*Pharmacologic:*

- Short-acting beta$_2$-agonists 30 min prior to exercise provides prevention in up to 90% of cases; also used for treatment of acute symptoms (albuterol, terbutaline)
- Long-acting beta$_2$-agonists 4 hs prior to exercise (salmeterol)
- Mast cell stabilizers 20 min prior to exercise may prevent symptoms in 70–80% of patients and have no side effects; may be effective in preventing late phase symptoms (Intal)
- Inhaled corticosteroids are helpful in patients with chronic asthma (Azmacort MDI 2 puffs bid–qid, Flovent MDI 88–220 mcg 2 puffs bid)
- Leukotriene modifiers may be effective in some cases (Accolate 20 mg po bid, Singulair 10 mg po qhs)
- Theophylline may be considered if there is inadequate response to standard prophylaxis
- Note: the USOC has banned all beta$_2$-agonists except albuterol, terbutaline, and salmeterol.

## 22.5 EXERCISE-INDUCED ANAPHYLAXIS

Phy Sportmed 1996;24(11):76; Allergy: Principles and Practice, 5th ed. St. Louis: Mosby Year Book, Inc, 1998; p 1109; Primary Care: Clin in Off Prac 1998;25:809; Clin Sport Med 1997;16:635

**Cause:**
- Exercise
- In many individuals there is an associated food such as celery, carrots, or wheat

**Epidem:**
- Rare condition
- More common in young people (mean 25 yrs)
- Female to male ratio is 2:1
- Two thirds of patients have a family history of atopy and 50% are themselves atopic

**Pathophys:** IgE mediated release of mast cell products leading to smooth muscle spasm, bronchospasm, mucosal edema and inflammation, and increased capillary permeability

**Sx:** Flushing sensation, pruritis, GI complaints such as vomiting, throat tightness or choking, headache

**Si:** Diffuse, large urticarial wheals (10–25 mm), angioedema, bronchospasm, syncope, hypotension

**Crs:**

- Symptoms typically begin soon after the start of exercise and resolve 30 min to 4 hs after cessation of activity
- Attacks do not occur with every exercise session
- Attacks are more common following meals and in warm or humid environments (Phy SportMed 1996;24(11):76)

**Cmplc:** Untreated cases may progress to shock and airway obstruction and are potentially life-threatening

**DiffDx:** Physical urticarias, exercise-induced anaphylaxis variant syndrome, cholinergic urticaria

**Lab:**

- Diagnosis is made from clinical history
- Laboratory tests are expensive and nonspecific making them rarely helpful
- Exercise challenge tests are nonspecific and can be risky

**Rx:**

- Acute treatment consists of immediate cessation of activity, movement to a cool place, and administration of injectable diphenhydramine
- In patients with symptoms of throat tightness, dyspnea, and lightheadedness, injectable epinephrine should be administered
- Prophylactic treatment has been largely unsuccessful and remains controversial
- Antihistamines have been shown in a few studies to decrease symptoms related to histamine release and remain the prophylaxis of choice
- Patient precautions: patients with exercise-induced anaphylaxis should wear a medical alert bracelet, carry epinephrine, never exercise alone, avoid known food precipitants prior to exercise, and exercise in cool time of day

## 22.6 CHOLINERGIC URTICARIA

Phy Sportmed 1996;24(11):76; Allergy: Principles and Practice, 5th ed. St. Louis: Mosby Year Book, 1998; p 1109; Primary Care: Clin in Off Prac 1998;25(4):809

**Cause:** Processes that raise the core body temperature by 0.5°C to 1.5°C (0.9°F to 2.7°F); specifically hot showers, anxiety, and exercise

**Epidem:** Rare condition; most common in young people

**Pathophys:** IgE mediated release of mast cell products

**Sx:** Headache, palpitations, abdominal cramps, diarrhea, sweating, flushing, lacrimation, salivation

**Si:**

- Small pruritic papules (2–4 mm) with surrounding macular erythema
- Bronchospasm and angioedema may occur in rare cases

**Crs:**

- Signs and symptoms develop 2–30 min following precipitant and last from 20–90 min
- Lesions appear first on upper thorax and neck but can spread distally to involve the entire body
- Hives can become confluent and resemble angioedema

**Cmplc:** Bronchospasm (clinically significant alteration in pulmonary function is unusual), angioedema, small risk of anaphylaxis, decreased fitness

**DiffDx:** Physical urticarias, exercise-induced anaphylaxis, exercise-induced anaphylaxis variant syndrome

**Lab:**

- Diagnosis made by clinical history
- Warming an extremity to raise core temperature by 0.50°C to 1.50°C is the most specific test
- Metacholine challenge test has only 50% sensitivity
- Laboratory tests are not helpful

**Rx:**

- Hydroxyzine hydrochloride is the antihistamine of choice for prophylaxis; doses of 100 mg to 200 mg/24 hr divided qid are usually sufficient
- Diphenhydramine or hydroxyzine may be used for treatment at time of flare-up
- Epinephrine may be prescribed due to small risk of anaphylaxis

# Index

Page numbers followed by f or t indicate figures or tables, respectively.

Abdominal pain, 262. *See also*
    Gastrointestinal symptoms
Abnormal liver function tests, 261
Acetabular labral tear, 132–133
Achilles tendinopathy, 187–188
    *vs.* retrocalcaneal bursitis, 201
Achilles tendon rupture, 181–183
Thompson squeeze test for, 181, 182f
Acromioclavicular osteoarthritis,
    65–66
    *vs.* rotator cuff tear, 63
Acromioclavicular separation, 57–58
    classification of, 57
    positive test for, 58
    *vs.* clavicle fracture, 59
Acute effort migraine, 208–209
Acute mountain sickness (AMS),
    21–22
Adductor tendon strain, 134–135
Adhesive capsulitis, 70–71
    *vs.* rotator cuff tendinopathy, 71
Amenorrhea, 248–249
Anabolic steroids, 40–41
    complications of, 41
    effects of, 40
Anaphylaxis, exercise-induced,
    278–279
Ankle injuries
    Achilles tendinopathy, 187–188
    Achilles tendon rupture, 181–183
    anterolateral soft-tissue
        impingement, 184

distal fibular stress fracture,
    186–187
osteochondral defect of the talus,
    180–181
peroneal tendon subluxation,
    177–178
posterior tibialis tendinopathy, 185
sinus tarsi syndrome, 186
sprain (*See* Ankle sprain)
Ankle sprain
    anterior drawer test for, 173, 174f
    grading of, 173
    high ankle, 178–180
    lateral ankle, 172–177
    rehabilitation phases for, 175–176
    *vs.* OCD of the talus, 181
    *vs.* sinus tarsi syndrome, 186
Anorexia nervosa, 251
Anterior apprehension test, for
    shoulder instability, 66, 67f
Anterior cruciate ligament (ACL),
    146–148
Anterior drawer test, for ankle sprain,
    173, 174f
Anterior shoulder dislocation, 59–61
Anterolateral impingement
    of ankle soft tissue, 184
    *vs.* OCD of the talus, 181
    *vs.* sinus tarsi syndrome, 186
Anxiety state, and use of stimulants, 44
Apley's compression test, for meniscus
    injuries, 151

Apley's scratch test, for adhesive capsulitis, 70
Apophysitis, 226–230
Arrhythmias
    and hypothermia, 33
    and use of stimulants, 44
Arthritis, *vs.* olecranon bursitis, 83
Asthma
    exercise-induced, 276–278
    heat exchange theory, 276
    water loss theory, 276
"Athlete's heart," *vs.* hypertrophic cardiomyopathy, 243
Avascular necrosis, and stress fracture, 7

Back pain. *See* Dioscogenic back pain; Low back pain, mechanical
Baker's cysts, 164–165
Bankart lesion, 60
    and shoulder instability, 68
Bennett's fracture, 101
Biceps tendonitis, 72–73
    positive tests for, 72
    Speed's test for, 72, 73f
Blisters, 189
Boxer's knuckle, 91
Bulimia, 251–252
Burner. *See* Transient brachial plexopathy
Bursitis
    calcific, 76
    greater trochanter, 137–138
    iliopectineal, 133–134
    ischiogluteal, 141–142
    olecranon, 82–84
    pes anserine, 163–164
    prepatellar, 162–163
    subacromial, 68–69
    trochanteric, 17
    *vs.* medial plica syndrome, 162
    *vs.* patellar tendinitis, 161
    *vs.* patellofemoral pain, 159

Buttocks pain
    ischiogluteal bursitis, 141–142
    piriformis syndrome, 140–141

Caffeine, as stimulant, 43–44, 45
Calcaneal stress fracture, 200
    *vs.* plantar fasciitis, 199
    *vs.* Sever's disease, 228
    *vs.* tarsal tunnel syndrome, 202
Calcific bursitis, 76
Cantu, return to play guidelines, 211, 212t
Carpal tunnel syndrome
    injection for, 13–14, 14f
    median nerve, 214–216
    Phalen's test for, 215, 215f
Cauda equina syndrome, 121, 122
Cellulitis, 269–270
    *vs.* olecranon bursitis, 83
Central slip avulsion, 92
Cerebral vascular accident, and hypothermia, 32
Cervical radiculopathy, 51–54
    *vs.* acromioclavicular osteoarthritis, 65
    *vs.* lateral tennis elbow, 78
    *vs.* medial epicondylitis, 80
Cervical spine
    degenerative disc disease, 50–51
    degenerative joint disease, 50–51
    instability, 55–56
    radiculopathy, 51–54
Cervical spondylosis, 50–51
Cervical sprain, 49–50
Cervical stenosis, *vs.* transient brachial plexopathy, 55
Cervical strain, 49–50
Chilblains, 26–27
Cholinergic urticaria, 280
Clavicle fracture, 58–59
    *vs.* acromioclavicular separation, 58
Coal miner's knee, 162–163
Cocaine, as stimulant, 43–44, 45
Cold urticaria, 27–28

Cold weather injuries, 25–34
Collateral ligament tears, 95
Colorado Medical Society
  grading system for concussions, 210–211, 211t
  return to play guidelines, 211, 212t
Compression fracture
  vs. discogenic back pain, 124
  vs. Scheuermann's kyphosis, 232
Compression test, for cervical radiculopathy, 52
Concussions, 210–212
  grading system for, 210–211, 211t
  return to play guidelines, 211, 212t
Coracoid fracture
  vs. acromioclavicular separation, 58
  vs. clavicle fracture, 59
Cord neurapraxia, and transient brachial plexopathy, 55
Corticosteroid injection therapy, principles of, 9–10
Crank test, for labral tear, 74
Creatine, 39–40
  complications from use of, 40
  ergogenic effects of, 39
Cyclist's palsy, 218

Deep vein thrombosis
  vs. frostbite, 29
  vs. tennis leg, 170
Degenerative joint disease
  and distal radius fracture, 110
  and lunate osteonecrosis, 109
  vs. deQuervain's tenosynovitis, 111
de Quervain's tenosynovitis, 111–112, 112f
  injection for, 10–11, 12f
  vs. scaphoid fracture, 106–107
Diarrhea, 268–269
Discogenic back pain, 123–125
  acute vs. subacute, 125
  distal neuro findings for, 124
  vs. mechanical low back pain, 122
  vs. sacroiliac dysfunction, 127

Diskitis, vs. discogenic back pain, 124
Disseminated intravascular coagulation
  and hyperthermia, 35
  and hypothermia, 32
Distal biceps tendon injury, 87–88
Distraction test, for cervical radiculopathy, 52
Dorsal impaction syndrome, 119
"Dowager's hump," 250
Drugs, banned by NCAA, 39

Eating disorders, in female athletes, 251–253
Elbow
  distal biceps tendon injury, 87–88
  fracture of, 84–85
  lateral epicondylitis, 77–79
  MCL instability, 85–86
  medial collateral ligament instability, 85–86
  medial epicondylitis, 79–81
  olecranon bursitis, 82–83
  osteochondritis dissicans of, 224–225
  PIN entrapment, 81–82
  tennis, 77–79
  traumatic injuries of, 84–85
Epicondylitis
  lateral, 77–79
  medial, 79–81
  vs. OCD of the elbow, 225
Erythropoietin, 43
Estrogen replacement, in female athletes, 249, 250–251
Exercise
  and overtraining, 272–273
  in pregnancy, 253–254
Exercise-associated amenorrhea (EAA), 248–249
Exercise-associated collapse (EAC), 235–238
Exercise-induced anaphylaxis, 278–279
Exercise-induced asthma, 276–278

Exercise-induced hematuria, 275
Exertional compartment syndrome
        (ECS), 168–170
    AAOS diagnostic standards for, 169
    *vs.* shin splints, 171
    *vs.* stress fractures, 167
Exertional migraine, 208–209
    prolonged, 209–210
Exertional rhabdomyolysis, 274–275
Extensor carpi ulnaris (ECU) tendinitis,
        113–114
Extensor hood, dislocation of, 91
Extensor tenosynovitis, *vs.* PIN
        entrapment, 82

FABER test, for sacroiliac dysfunction,
        126, 126f
Female athletes
    eating disorders in, 251–253
    and exercise-associated amniorrhea,
        248–249
    osteoporosis in, 250–251
    and pregnancy, 253–254
    and stress fractures, 6
Femoral head avascular necrosis,
        131–132
Femoral stress fracture, 130–131
Fifth metatarsal fracture, 196–197
Finkelstein's test, for DeQuervain's
        tenosynovitis, 111, 112f
Flexor carpi ulnaris, 114
Flexor digitorum, 114
Flexor tenosynovitis, 114–115
Football finger, 90–91
Foot injuries
    blisters, 189
    forefoot, 190–197
    hindfoot, 199–203
    metatarsal fractures, 195–197
    midfoot, 197–199
    nails, 190
    sesamoid problems, 192–193
    tarsal fracture, 197–198
    turftoe, 191

Fracture
    ankle, 186–187
    clavicle, 58–59
    elbow, 84–85
    foot, 186–187
    hand, 97–101
    Lisfranc, 198–199
    Salter-Harris, 232–234
    wrist, 106–110
Freiberg's infarction, 194
Frostbite, 28–30
    degrees of, 28–29
Frostnip, 28, 30

Gamekeeper's thumb, 96–97
Gastrointestinal bleeding, 259–261
Gastrointestinal symptoms
    lower, 257–259
    upper, 255–257
Glasgow Coma Scale, 211
Golfer's elbow, 79–81
"Goose foot sign," 116
Greater trochanter bursitis, 137–138
Guillain-Barré, 268

Hallux rigidus, 192
Hallux valgus, 190–191
Hand dislocations
    DIP joint, 101–102
    MCP, 104–105
    PIP dorsal, 102–103
    PIP palmar, 103–104
Hand fractures
    Bennett's, 101
    CMC fracture dislocation, 101
    metacarpal, 99–100
    middle phalangeal, 97–98
    PIP fracture dislocation, 98
    proximal phalangeal, 99
Hand ligament injuries
    collateral tears, 94
    gamekeeper's thumb, 96–97
    PIP volar plate rupture, 95
    skier's thumb, 96–97

Hand tendon injuries
  central slip avulsion, 92
  dislocation of extensor hood, 91
  Jersey finger, 90–91
  mallet finger, 89–90
  trigger finger, 93
Hawkin's impingement sign, 62, 64f, 69
Headaches
  benign exertional, 207
  and concussions, 210
  migraines, 208–210
  weightlifter's, 208
Heat cramps, 34, 35, 36
Heat exhaustion, 35, 36
Heat injuries, 34–37
Heat stroke, 35, 36
Heat syncope, 34, 35, 36
Heel injuries, 199–201
Hematuria, exercise-induced, 275
Hepatic injury, 261
Herniated disc
  vs. cervical spondylosis, 51
  vs. transient brachial plexopathy, 55
Herniated nucleus pulposus (HNP), 123–125
Herpes, 270–271
High-altitude cerebral edema (HACE), 23–25
  and acute mountain sickness, 22
High-altitude injuries, 21–25
High-altitude pulmonary edema (HAPE), and acute mountain sickness, 22, 23
Hill Sachs lesion, 60
  and shoulder instability, 68
Hip, toxic synovitis of, 232
Hip injury
  acetabular labral tear, 132–133
  adductor tendon strain, 134–135
  femoral head avascular necrosis, 131–132
  femoral stress fracture, 130–131
  greater trochanter bursitis, 137–138
  hip pointer, 139–140
  iliopectineal bursitis, 133–134
  iliopsoas tendon strain, 135
  osteitis pubis, 136
Hip pointer, 139–140
Housemaid's knee, 162–163
Human growth hormone, 41–42
  complications from use of, 42
  ergogenic effects of, 42
Hypertension, 238–241
  classification of, 239t, 241
  lifestyle modification for, 240
  and restriction from sports, 241, 242t
Hyperthermia, 34–37
  and disseminated intravascular coagulation, 35
  malignant, 36
Hypertrophic cardiomyopathy (HCM), 241–244
  vs. exercise-associated collapse, 237
Hypothermia, 30–34
  and arrhythmias, 33
  and frostbite, 32
  vs. rigor mortis, 32
Hypoxia
  and acute mountain sickness (AMS), 21
  and high-altitude cerebral edema, 23–25
  and high-altitude pulmonary edema, 23–25

Ice water immersion test, 28
Iliopectineal bursitis, 133–134
Iliopsoas tendon strain, 135
Iliotibial band friction syndrome (ITBFS), 165–166
Immersion foot, 25–26
Impingement, 68–69
  Hawkin's sign, 62, 64f, 69
  Neer sign, 69
  positive tests for, 69
  test, 62, 64f

Impingement (*cont.*)
  *vs.* calcific bursitis, 76
  *vs.* rotator cuff tear, 63
  *vs.* rotator cuff tendinopathy, 71
Infectious diseases, 263–269
  and overtraining, 273
Infectious mononucleosis (IM),
    267–268
  *vs.* upper respiratory infection,
    264
Inflammatory sacroiliitis, *vs.* sacroiliac
    dysfunction, 127
Injection therapy
  for carpal tunnel syndrome, 12–14,
    14f
  corticosteroid, principles of, 9–10
  for de Quervain's tenosynovitis,
    10–11, 12f
  for intra-articular knee, 18, 19f
  for plantar fascia, 19–20
  for subacromial space, 16–17, 16f
  for tennis elbow, 15, 15f
  for triangular fibrocartilage complex
    (TFCC), 12–13, 13f
  for trigger finger, 10, 11f
  for trochanteric bursitis, 17
Intra-articular knee, injection for, 18,
    19f
Intracranial hemorrhage, 213–214
Ischemic limb, *vs.* chilblains, 27
Ischial bursitis, *vs.* discogenic back
    pain, 124
Ischiogluteal bursitis, 141–142

Jersey finger, 90–91
Jogger's migraine, 209–210

Kienböck's disease, 108–109
Knee, osteochondritis dessicans of,
    222–224
Knee injuries
  anterior cruciate ligament, 146–148
  collateral ligament, 155–158
  meniscal tear, 150–151

patellar dislocation, 152–154
patellar tendon rupture, 154–155
posterior cruciate injuries, 148–150
Knee pain
  bursitis, 162–164
  ITB friction syndrome, 165–166
  medial plica syndrome, 161–162
  patellofemoral, 158
  popliteal cysts, 164–165
  tendinitis, 160–161

Labral tear, 74, 76
  positive tests for, 74, 75f
  *vs.* shoulder instability, 68
Lachman test, for anterior cruciate
    ligament, 147, 147f
Lateral ankle sprain, 172–177
Lateral collateral ligament injury,
    157–158
Lateral epicondylitis, 77–79
  *vs.* PIN entrapment, 81–82
Lateral tennis elbow, 77–79
Leg
  exertional compartment syndrome,
    168–169
  fascial compartments of, 168t
  medial tibial stress syndrome, 171
  stress fractures, 167–168
  tennis, 170
Legg-Calvé-Perthes (LCP) disease,
    231
  *vs.* SCFE, 230
Ligamentous sprain, 49–50
Lisfranc dislocation, 198–199
Lisfranc fracture, 198–199
Lisfranc joint injury, *vs.* metatarsal
    fracture, 195
Little League elbow, 228–230
  *vs.* OCD of the elbow, 225
Liver, injury of, 261
Liver function tests, 261
Long QT syndrome (LQTS), 247
  *vs.* exercise-associated collapse,
    237

Low back pain, mechanical
    acute *vs.* subacute, 122
    *vs.* discogenic back pain, 124
Lumbar spinal stenosis, 127–129

Maisonneuve's fracture, 179
Malignant hyperthermia, 36
Mallet finger, 89–90
McMurray's test, 150
Medial collateral ligament (MCL)
    injury, 155–156
    instability, 85–86
Medial elbow apophysitis, 228–230
Medial epicondylitis, 79–81
Medial plica syndrome, 161–162
Medial tibial stress syndrome (MTSS),
    171
Meniscus injuries, 150–151
    *vs.* ACL injury, 148
    *vs.* OCD of the knee, 223
    *vs.* posterior cruciate injury, 149
Metastatic disease, *vs.* lumbar spinal
    stenosis, 128
Metatarsal fracture, 195
    *vs.* Lisfranc joint injury, 198
Metatarsal stress fracture, 196
    *vs.* Freiberg's infarction, 194
Migraine
    acute effort, 208–209
    exertional, 208–209
    jogger's, 209–210
    prolonged exertional, 209–210
"Milking" sign, 86
Mitral valve prolapse (MVP), 245–247
    *vs.* exercise-associated collapse, 237
Mononucleosis, infectious, 267–268
Monteggia's fracture, 81
Morton's neuroma, *vs.* Freiberg's
    infarction, 193–194
Myocarditis, 244–245
    *vs.* exercise-associated collapse,
    237
Myofascial neck pain, 49–50
Myositis ossificans, 144

NCAA, drugs banned by, 38
Neck strain, 49–50
Neer impingement sign, 69
Neuropsychometric testing, for
    concussions, 211
Nirschl's Pain Phase Scale, 4
Nutrition. *See also* Eating disorders, in
        female athletes
    guidelines for optimum performance,
        38t
    U.S. government guidelines for, 38

Ober's test
    for greater trochanter bursitis, 137,
        138f
    for iliotibial band friction syndrome,
        166
Olecranon bursitis, 82–84
Osgood-Schlatter disease (OSD), 226
    *vs.* Sinding-Larsen-Johansson, 227
Osteitis pubis, 136
Osteoarthritis, 50–51
    acromioclavicular, 65–66
    *vs.* rotator cuff tear, 63
    *vs.* tendinosis, 71
Osteochondral defect (OCD), of the
    talus, 180–181
Osteochondritis dessicans (OCD)
    of the elbow, 224–225
    of the knee, 222–224
Osteoid osteoma, *vs.* acromioclavicular
    osteoarthritis, 65
Osteolysis, *vs.* acromioclavicular
    separation, 58
Osteoporosis, in female athletes,
    250–251
Os trigonum syndrome, 203
Otitis media, 265
Overtraining, 272–273
Overuse injuries, 3–6

Pancreatitis, *vs.* mechanical low back
    pain, 122
Panner's disease, 224–225

Patellar apprehension test, 152, 153f
Patellar dislocation, 152–154
  *vs.* ACL injury, 146–148
  *vs.* posterior cruciate injury, 149
Patellar grind test, 159
Patellar subluxation, 152–154
Patellar tendinitis
  *vs.* Osgood-Schlatter disease, 226
  *vs.* patellofemoral pain, 159
Patellar tendon rupture, 154–155
Patellofemoral pain, 158–160
Peripheral nerve injury, *vs.* cervical
      radiculopathy, 53
Peritendonitis, *vs.* Achilles
      tendinopathy, 187
Pernio, 26–27
Peroneal tendon subluxation, 177–178
Pes anserine bursitis, 163–164
Phalangeal fractures, 195
Phalen's test, for carpal tunnel
      syndrome, 215, 215f
Pheochromocytoma, *vs.* stimulants, 44
PIP volar plate rupture, 95
Piriformis syndrome, 140–141
Pitcher's elbow, 79–81
Plantar fasciitis, 199–200
  injection for, 19–20, 20f
  *vs.* calcaneal stress fracture, 200
  *vs.* Sever's disease, 228
Pneumonia, 266–267
Popliteal cysts, 164–165
Positive cotton test, for high ankle
      sprain, 178, 179f
Positive squeeze test
  for Achilles tendon rupture, 181,
      182f
  for high ankle sprain, 178
Posterior cruciate injuries, 148–150
Posterior dislocation test, for shoulder
      instability, 67
Posterior interosseous nerve (PIN)
      entrapment, 81–82
  *vs.* cervical radiculopathy, 78
Posterior tibialis tendinopathy, 185

Posterior tibialis tendon rupture, 183
Pregnancy, exercise in, 253–254
Prepatellar bursitis, 162–163
Pronator syndrome, 216–217
Pyelonephritis, *vs.* mechanical low
      back pain, 122
Pyriformis syndrome, *vs.* discogenic
      back pain, 124

Quadriceps tendon rupture, 154–155
Quadriparesis, and cervical
      spondylosis, 50

Radial head fracture, *vs.* cervical
      radiculopathy, 78
Radial nerve neuropathy, 218
Radial tunnel syndrome, 81–82, 218
Raynaud's disease, *vs.* chilblains, 27
Refractory ventricular fibrillation, and
      hypothermia, 32
Relocation test, for shoulder
      instability, 67
Retrocalcaneal bursitis, 201
  *vs.* Achilles tendinopathy, 187
  *vs.* os trigonum syndrome, 203
Retropatellar knee pain, 158–160
  *vs.* OCD of the knee, 223
Rhabdomyolysis
  exertional, 274–275
  and hyperthermia, 35
Ring worm, 271
"Ripped fuel," as stimulant, 43
Rockwood technique, for anterior
      shoulder dislocation, 60
Rotator cuff tear, 61–65
  positive test for, 62
  *vs.* acromioclavicular separation, 58
  *vs.* adhesive capsulitis, 70
  *vs.* labral tear, 74
Rotator cuff tendinopathy, 71–72
  *vs.* calcific bursitis, 76
  *vs.* labral tear, 74
  *vs.* rotator cuff tear, 63
  *vs.* shoulder instability, 68

Sacroiliac (SI) dysfunction, 125–126
 FABER test for, 126, 126f
 *vs.* mechanical low back pain, 122
Salter-Harris fractures, 232–234
 classification of, 233, 233f
Scaphoid fracture, 106–107
 *vs.* de Quervain's tenosynovitis, 111
Scapholunate (SL) dissociation,
  116–117
Scheuermann's kyphosis, 221–222
 *vs.* spondylolysis, 219
Sciatica, 123–125
"Scotty dog," 219
Second impact syndrome, 213
Sesamoiditis, 192–193
 *vs.* hallux rigidus, 192
Sesamoid stress fracture, 193
Sever's disease, 227–228
Shin splints, 171
Shock, and hyperthermia, 36
Shoulder, frozen, 70–71
Shoulder injuries
 acromioclavicular osteoarthritis,
   65–66
 acromioclavicular separation,
   57–58
 biceps tendonitis, 72–73
 calcific bursitis, 76
 clavicle fracture, 58–59
 dislocation, 59–61
 frozen shoulder, 70–71
 impingement, 68
 labral tear, 74–76
 rotator cuff tear, 61–65
 rotator cuff tendinopathy, 71–72
Shoulder instability, 66–68
 anterior apprehension test for, 66,
   67f
 positive tests for, 66–68
 posterior dislocation test for, 67
 relocation test for, 67
Side stitch, 262
Sinding-Larsen-Johansson (SLJ)
  disease, 227

Sinusitis, 266
 *vs.* upper respiratory infection, 264
Sinus tarsi syndrome, 186
Skiers' thumb, 96–97
Skin infections, 269–271
SLAPrehension test, for labral tear, 74,
  75f
Slipped capital femoral epiphysis
  (SCFE), 230–231
 *vs.* Legg-Calvé-Perthes (LCP) disease,
   230–231
 *vs.* toxic synovitis of the hip, 232
Snapping hip syndrome, 139
Speed's test, for biceps tendonitis, 72,
  73f
Spinal stenosis, 50–51
Spondylolisthesis, 220–221
Spondylolysis, 219–220
Sports, static *vs.* dynamic classification
  of, 242t
Sprain
 ankle, 172–180
 cervical, 49–50
 elbow, 84–85
Spurling's test, 52, 53f
Sternoclavicular joint subluxation,
  *vs.* clavicle fracture, 59
Steroids. *See* Anabolic steroids
Stimson technique, for anterior
  shoulder dislocation, 60
Stimulants, 43–45
 ergogenic effects of, 44
Stinger. *See* Transient brachial
  plexopathy
Strain
 adductor tendon, 134–135
 cervical, 49–50
 elbow, 84–85
 iliopsoas tendon, 135
 neck, 49–50
 thigh muscle, 142–143
Stress fracture, 6–8
 calcaneal, 200
 distal fibular, 186–187

Stress fracture (*cont.*)
  femoral, 130–131
  foot, 195–196
  leg, 167–168
Subacromial bursitis, 68–69
Subacromial space, injection for,
    16–17, 16f
Subluxation, patellar, 152–154
Subungual hematoma, 190
Sudden death
  and hypertrophic cardiomyopathy,
    243
  and long QT syndrome, 47
  and mitral valve prolapse, 246
  and myocarditis, 244
  and use of stimulants, 44
Supinator syndrome, 81–82
Supraspinatus strength test, 62, 63f
Syncope, 235–238
  neurocardiogenic, 235–236
Syndesmosis injury, 178–179
  *vs.* ankle sprain, 179
Synovitis, toxic, 232
  *vs.* SCFE, 230

Tarsal navicular stress fracture, *vs.*
    posterior tibialis tendinopathy,
    185
Tarsal stress fracture, 197–198
Tarsal tunnel syndrome, 201–202
  *vs.* calcaneal stress fracture, 200
  *vs.* plantar fasciitis, 199
  *vs.* posterior tibialis tendinopathy,
    185
  *vs.* retrocalcaneal bursitis, 201
Tendinitis, 76
  biceps, 72–73
  *vs.* metatarsal fracture, 195, 196
  *vs.* olecranon bursitis, 83
  patellar, 160–161
  *vs.* sesamoiditis, 193
Tendinosis, *vs.* adhesive capsulitis,
    71
Tendonitis. *See* Tendinitis

Tennis elbow
  injection for, 15, 15f
  lateral, 77–79
Tennis leg, 170
Thigh
  avulsion injuries, 145
  muscle contusions, 143–144
  muscle strains, 142–143
  myositis ossificans, 144
Thompson squeeze test, for Achilles
    tendon rupture, 181, 182f
Thoracic outlet syndrome, *vs.* cervical
    radiculopathy, 53
Tinea, 271
Toe injuries, 190–197
Training, excessive, 272–273
Transient brachial plexopathy, 54–55
  *vs.* spinal spondylosis, 51
Traumatic brain injury (TBI)
  concussions, 210–212
  intracranial hemorrhage, 213–214
  second impact syndrome, 213
Trench foot, 25
Triangular fibrocartilage complex
    (TFCC)
  injection for, 12–13, 13f
  tear, 117–118
Trigger finger, 93
  injection for, 10, 11f
Trochanteric bursitis, injection for, 17
Turf toe, 191
  *vs.* hallux rigidus, 192

Ulnar collateral ligament sprain
classes of, 96
  *vs.* medial epicondylitis, 80
Ulnar nerve neuropathy, 217–218
Upper respiratory infection (URI),
    264
Urticaria, cold, 27–28

Valgus stress test, for medial collateral
    ligament injury, 155
Viral syndrome, 263

Weaver's bottom, 141–142
Weightlifter's headache, 208
Weight loss, and use of stimulants, 44
Whiplash, 49–50
Wrist fractures
  distal radius, 109–110
  hamate, 107
  lunate osteonecrosis, 108–109
  scaphoid, 106–107

Wrist ganglion, 119–120
Wrist tendon injuries
  common extensor tenosynovitis,
    115–116
  de Quervain's tenosynovitis,
    111–112, 112f
  extensor carpi ulnaris, 113–114
  flexor tenosynovitis, 114–115
  intersection syndrome, 112–113